MAKING THE PROZAC DECISION

A GUIDE TO ANTIDEPRESSANTS

Newly Revised Third Edition

By Carol Ann Turkington
and Eliot F. Kaplan, M.D.

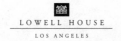

LOWELL HOUSE
LOS ANGELES

CONTEMPORARY BOOKS
CHICAGO

RC
537
.T87
1997

Library of Congress Cataloging-in-Publication Data
Turkington, Carol
Making the prozac decision : a guide to antidepressants / Carol Turkington, with Eliot F. Kaplan.
    p.   cm.
Includes bibliographical references and index.
ISBN 1-56565-153-7
1. Depression, Mental—Chemotherapy. 2. Depression, Mental—Popular works.
3. Antidepressants. I. Kaplan, Eliot F. II Title.
RC537.T87   1994
616.85'27061—dc20   94-5356
                                                                                      CIP

Lowell House
2020 Avenue of the Stars, Suite 300
Los Angeles, California 90067

Publisher: Jack Artenstein
Associate Publisher, Lowell House Adult: Bud Sperry
Project Editor: Peter Hoffman
Text design: Frank Loose Design, Portland, Oregon

Manufactured in the United States of America

10   9   8   7   6   5   4   3   2   1

DEDICATION

To my old friends Elaine and Jill, who have known the kingdom of night.

—*Carol Ann Turkington*

To all those people thinking about pursuing treatment, as well as those currently in treatment for depression.

—*Eliot F. Kaplan, M.D.*

> *"No one is capable of gratitude as one who has emerged from the kingdom of night."*
>
> —*Elie Wiesel*

The authors caution readers not to use this book exclusively to diagnose themselves or others. Outlines of symptoms are presented here to suggest the many faces that depression may wear. If you believe you or someone you care about may be depressed, it's imperative to get help from a qualified mental health professional.

The authors have tried to ensure that all information in this book concerning drug dosages, schedules, and treatments is accurate at the time of publication and consistent with the standards set by the U.S. Food and Drug Administration and the general medical community. However, as medical research advances, therapeutic standards may change.

For this reason and because individual cases may differ, we strongly recommend that you follow the advice of a physician directly involved in your care or the care of a family member.

CONTENTS

ACKNOWLEDGMENTS

This book would not have been possible without the cooperation of countless women and men whose generosity of spirit contributed to *Making the Prozac Decision*. My heartfelt thanks to these people who so willingly shared their deeply personal stories of depression so that others might learn from their experiences. Special thanks for valuable referrals given by Dr. Jack Sturgis, Gail Novick, Jill Selleck, Elaine Bernarding and Barbara Turkington, and to Ross, for all the inside scoops.

Thanks also to a wide variety of psychiatric experts who have discussed their personal approach, to antidepressant therapy, and to the staffs of the American Psychological Association, American Psychiatric Association, the National Institutes of Health, and the medical libraries of the National Library of Medicine, Hershey Medical Center, and the University of Pennsylvania Medical Center. Thanks also to Steve Berchem at Pharmaceutical Research and Manufacturers of America and to staffers at Eli Lilly, Astra USA, Bristol-Myers, Burroughs Wellcome, Ciba-Geigy, Hoffmann-LaRoche, Pfizer, SmithKline Beecham, and Solvay Pharmaceuticals.

Finally, my thanks to my agent Bert Holtje, for all his help; to Peter Hoffman for tireless support and terrific editing, and most of all, to Michael and to Kara, who have so generously shared me with my computer.

—*Carol Ann Turkington*

I would like to thank Roseann, my best friend and wife (and an excellent nurse psychotherapist), for her love and support.

I appreciate the thorough, broad-based training that I had at Jefferson Medical College and then in my psychiatry residency at Thomas Jefferson University Hospital in Philadelphia, which helped me to become the psychiatrist I am today.

I would like to thank my children, Melanie and Jason, for their love and patience while I worked on this book.

—*Eliot F. Kaplan, M.D.*

FOREWORD

I have been gratified by the positive response to *Making the Prozac Decision*. Shedding light on the appropriate use of antidepressants is the central focus of this book, and as the 1990s proceed, the prescription of antidepressant medication consumes an increasing proportion of the practicing psychiatrist's time and effort. With the increasing development of managed care in recent years, psychiatrists are called on less frequently to provide psychotherapy (now usually conducted by psychologists, social workers, and nurse psychotherapists) and more frequently to prescribe psychiatric drugs. My own practice is not immune to this trend.

There seems to be an increasing public acceptance of the "reality" of depression and the need for treatment. The selective serotonin reuptake inhibitors (SSRIs) are widely prescribed by primary care physicians as well as psychiatrists. I have seen an increase in interest and questions about alternative approaches as well—including acupuncture, Thought Field Therapy, Eye Movement Desensitization Reprocessing (EMDR), and herbal medications. (For example, I'll be discussing St. John's wort later in the book).

While the prescription of antidepressant medication in 1997 is as much art as science, I believe that any physician prescribing these drugs should have an organized, step by step approach should the first (or second or third) medication fail to help. Such an approach is often called a *decision tree*.

Typically, the first drug of choice to treat depression is an SSRI such as Prozac, Zoloft, or Paxil; if that doesn't relieve the person's depression, following is how I would proceed to the next drug of choice, and the next, and so on along my own decision tree:

Step 1. SSRI: Either Prozac, Zoloft, or Paxil

Step 2. *If no sexual dysfunction:*
different SSRI of above three

If there is sexual dysfunction:
with anxiety: Serzone
no anxiety: Wellbutrin

Step 3. Effexor

Step 4. Remeron

Step 5. tricyclic antidepressant (Pamelor or Norpramin)

Step 6. monoamine oxidase inhibitor (Nardil or Parnate)

Step 7. herbal preparation (St. John's wort)

Step 8. *Very rarely:*
electroconvulsive treatment (ECT)

A patient who responds partially to one of the above antidepressants often benefits from the addition of another drug, such as BuSpar, lithium, or Ritalin, for example. Obviously, there are exceptions and deviations from the decision tree—that's where the art comes in.

What's important for you to understand is that the treatment of depression is typically *very* successful—*if* you keep trying if the first drug combination doesn't work. Sometimes persistence is needed.

—*Eliot F. Kaplan, M.D.*
June 1997

I completed my training in 1984, before the introduction of the newer antidepressants: the selective serotonin reuptake inhibitors (Prozac, Zoloft, and Paxil), Wellbutrin, and Effexor. Most of my career has been in the private practice of psychiatry, seeing outpatients in my office, working with patients in a 300-bed community hospital, treating patients on the mental health unit there, and doing consulting work with patients admitted medically. I have treated thousands of depressed patients (both male and female from their teens to their nineties), with symptoms ranging from mild adjustment problems to suicidal thoughts and/or psychosis. The work I have done is clinical, involving treatment rather than research or teaching.

My approach to treatment has typically started with patient education, including a summary of their situation, diagnosis, treatment options (with pros and cons), and prognosis. I try to help patients reach their goals, if that's feasible. I believe it's important to provide a trusting environment in which patients can discuss what is important to them. My approach is eclectic, using elements of insight, supportive and behavioral therapies, and antidepressant medication if needed.

It is important to realize that depression is a symptom of an illness, not a manifestation of moral or spiritual weakness. Depressive illness is akin to some medical problems with physiological bases that are affected by situational and temperamental factors such as hypertension, headache, diabetes mellitus, and irritable bowel syndrome. There are several types of depressive illness of varying severity, including adjustment disorder with depressed mood, dysthymia, major depressive episode, and bipolar disorder (manic-depressive illness). Before you embark on treatment for depression, it's important to have an evaluation to rule out any medical problems that could be causing or aggravating the depression.

It is worth considering what antidepressant medications do. They correct neurotransmitter problems in the brain that are associated with depression. About 80 percent of the time, they are extremely effective in helping with depression and the concomitant crying, sleep and appetite disturbances, suicidal ideas, feelings of hopelessness, concentration problems, lack of energy and interest, and so on. These medications work for as long as they're taken; they're a symptomatic treatment. The reason a person continues to do well after the antidepressant medication is stopped is that the depression has run its course.

Antidepressant medications work fairly quickly, sometimes within a few weeks, rather than the months that are typically needed in a purely psychotherapeutic approach. I've seen patients who have been in psychotherapy elsewhere for years without much benefit. When I've tried antidepressant medications in those patients, the results have often been excellent. Antidepressant medications can complement psychotherapy. The better a person feels, the more he or she can participate in the treatment. Patients with severe depression can be so preoccupied and withdrawn that they can't engage in psychotherapy at all until they've had some symptom relief.

It is also important to realize what antidepressant medications *don't* do. In my opinion, they do *not* change personality; they treat depression. Depression can cause withdrawal, poor self-esteem, timidity, quietness, and lack of enthusiasm. Treatment frees the person to be himself or herself. The depression may have persisted for years with an insidious onset, complicating and obscuring the pervasiveness of the symptoms. Antidepressant medications are not addictive. Antidepressant medications do not turn people into zombies. Antidepressant medications do not cure depression. They are part of a treatment regimen.

The various types of antidepressant medications will be explored in this book. In my practice, the selective serotonin reuptake inhibitors (SSRIs) are usually my first choice in treating depression. All three (Prozac, Zoloft, and Paxil) work well, and are well-tolerated. They are safe in overdose and typically can be taken in a single daily dose. The unfortunate and often inaccurate media representation of Prozac has frightened many people to the point where patients and/or their families won't let me prescribe it. My educational efforts are often futile. I have certainly seen many wonderful responses to Prozac. Zoloft is the SSRI that I most often prescribe. Although I sometimes have to adjust the dosage, I have found it to have the fewest side effects of the three.

Paxil is the most sedating of the SSRIs, and when patients are suffering with insomnia, Paxil given at bedtime can be the answer. Wellbutrin, which has few side effects but needs to be taken two or three times a day, is usually my second choice. If a person can't tolerate the SSRIs or doesn't benefit from them, I'll prescribe Wellbutrin. My third choice is usually one of the tricyclic antidepressants (TCAs), nortriptyline or desipramine. The TCAs are the oldest category of antidepressants and have more side effects than the newer medications. However, checking blood levels gives reliable information about dosage needs. (The newer antidepressants do not have meaningful blood levels.)

After these three choices, I'll try one of the other agents—trazodone, maprotiline, one of the monoamine oxidase inhibitors (MAOIs), or Effexor. Infrequently, combinations of medications are needed.

A commonly asked question is "How long should I take this antidepressant?" For a major depressive episode, the medication is typically continued for about six months before a reduction is tried. If the symptoms recur, the original dosage is resumed. For a dysthymia, a mild but persistent form of depression, the reduction is tried after a year. I warn patients that the depression may reappear in the future. If that happens, early resumption of treatment is advisable. Typically, restarting a medication that worked in the past will prove successful. In rare situations, the recommendation is lifelong medication.

In summary, depressive illnesses deserve prompt, aggressive therapy. Without treatment, depression can end in suicide. At the very least, depression affects the quality of life of those suffering from it.

To the millions of people plagued by depression: I encourage you to take the first step by getting a thorough psychiatric evaluation. You and your psychiatrist can work together to make the decisions that are best for you. For most, treatment does work.

—*Eliot F. Kaplan, M.D.*

INTRODUCTION

> *"I was depressed my entire life. I kept going to doctors and telling them I didn't feel right. I felt icky. Crummy. Yucky. Once I started taking antidepressants, I realized I never felt like this in my entire life. It's called well-being."*
>
> —*Susan, 38*

To be depressed is to live with a sense of nothingness. People who are depressed say they feel numb, they feel empty, they feel invisible. Incredibly, two out of every ten Americans live their lives teetering on the edge of such an abyss, without any expectation that things will ever get better.

Who are they? They're people like Violet, a 38-year-old South Carolina nurse who developed depression following a liver transplant. "When I became depressed, I had no emotions at all," she recalls. "I always delighted at spring in South Carolina. But when I was depressed, I could look at the blooms and know it was beautiful, *but I had no sensory enjoyment of it.* I had my cat for 10 years, but when she died I didn't feel anything. Even as I was burying her, I felt nothing."

For four months, Violet hid her depression. "I really thought it was my fault," she says. "I thought my depression was an inappropriate response to receiving a life-saving organ. It wasn't okay to be feeling this way." When she finally confessed her depression to a psychiatrist, she was immediately given Prozac.

Within a few weeks, her depression began to lift. "It wasn't that I was suddenly effusive," Violet recalls. "I just started *feeling* again. Then one day, I came back from the store with extra supplies of dishwashing detergent and toothpaste, and I realized I was going to live. On a very deep level, I knew I would be washing my dishes and brushing my teeth two weeks from now. To me, it was a sign that I was getting better."

Perhaps you know someone like Violet—or maybe you feel this way yourself. You may have heard glowing reports about Prozac, and now you're wondering if it's really possible for any drug to work that well. Or you may have heard about Zoloft, Effexor, Luvox—some of the newer antidepressants that have been crowding Prozac off the front pages lately.

On the other hand, perhaps you've heard rumors of drug-induced suicide, the accusation by some of these drugs may be changing not just how they feel but *who they are*.

Are these drugs some sort of new salvation for depressed people, or is there a price to pay for the elimination of misery? Some experts warn that these medications are the new fad drug of the '90s, that they promise to pave the way to nirvana for nondepressed people.

Psychiatrist Richard Metzner is a UCLA associate professor of psychiatry who says he's prescribed Prozac for hundreds of patients in the past six years and doesn't know of one who's experienced the kind of miraculous personality change that's being discussed so much on talk shows and in the media. The notion of Prozac as a personality pill was characterized by psychiatrist Peter Kramer, author of the best-seller *Listening to Prozac,* who described its effects as cosmetic, not therapeutic. But Metzner argues that Prozac returns the working of the chemical composition of the brain to normal—and that, he says, is far from cosmetic.

Sorting out the pros and cons of antidepressant therapy can be a daunting task. But given the numbers of Americans currently taking these drugs, it's an important one. *Making the Prozac Decision* provides the latest information on antidepressants and the possible risks and benefits of these drugs. You'll also hear from men and women who've used all sorts of drugs, some of which worked and some of which didn't.

Making the Prozac Decision can help you understand what depression is and how it can be treated. Sidebars provide additional information on side effects and possible drug interactions. You'll learn how to handle depression, how to tell if someone's depressed or suicidal, and how to join an experimental antidepressant study.

Making the Prozac Decision will help you understand the differences between antidepressants, as well as the potential side effects, problems, and benefits of each drug.

You'll also find an extensive list of organizations to contact for further information.

Antidepressant therapy involves complex medical decisions between you and your doctor. It's vital that you understand the benefits and risks of this type of treatment, because depression is not a simple problem. If you get a prescription for an antidepressant and it's just not helping or you can't tolerate the side effects, be honest about it. You need to form a working alliance with your doctor and to understand that there is no shame in getting help. If you're not getting relief with a particular antidepressant, it's not your fault.

There's no miracle antidepressant that works for everybody, every time. If you're taking an antidepressant drug now, is it the best choice for you? Do you fully understand the side effects of the drugs you're taking? If one antidepressant isn't working, is your doctor willing to find one that does?

"If the first drug doesn't work, don't give up," cautions psychiatrist Andy Myerson of North Carolina. "You need to go to a psychiatrist who won't judge you. Some doctors tend to say, `If you don't get better, it's your fault.' But I've found that it's important to keep trying different antidepressants, because the tenth drug might work. Keep calling your doctor if you can't stand the side effects. If he or she won't help you, go to someone else."

1
WHAT IS DEPRESSION?

"When I was a teenager, it was as if one day a curtain dropped and I fell into the deepest, darkest abyss. That's what I've been battling for more than 25 years. My depression interfered with every conceivable part of my life."

—Alison, 47

Eleanor, 40, is a bright, attractive, well-educated Denver stockbroker who has struggled with feelings of overwhelming sadness for at least 25 years. "I can't remember when I wasn't depressed," she says today. Although her depression probably began in childhood, it was in college that she realized something was very wrong.

"I tried Rolfing, transactional analysis, meditation. I cut out coffee, smoking, and alcohol. I went on vegetarian diets, juice diets, and fasts. I kept trying all these alternative therapies because I thought that something should help the way I felt."

How she felt, she says, was miserable. "My body ached, the way you feel right before you get the flu—lethargic and hurting. That's why I smoked dope and drank alcohol; I was trying anything to feel better. But nothing worked." Then, in her mid-thirties Eleanor was injured in a car accident, and her depression deepened.

"I cried all day long. I would cry at every TV show—even 'Gunsmoke' and 'I Love Lucy'," she recalls. "I kept asking doctors why I was so depressed." Eleanor's psychologist finally became angry: "One day she snapped at me," Eleanor recalls, "and she said, 'Do you want me to send you to a psychiatrist so you can *take pills?* She said it as if taking pills was a moral failure."

After another six months of fruitless talk therapy, Eleanor finally did go to see a psychiatrist, who did indeed prescribe an antidepressant for her depression—one of the most serious cases he said he'd ever seen. After her doctor tried three or four different medications, Eleanor's depression finally responded to a combination of Paxil and lithium.

"I feel as if I've been ripped off my entire life because I was depressed for so long," Eleanor says. "Now I have my sense of humor back. I feel great. I feel *normal.*"

Many people have stories similar to Eleanor's. Depression is far more common than most people realize: Two out of every ten of us are clinically depressed. As many as 23 percent of all adult women have had one major depressive episode in their lifetime.

The tragedy is that although so many people are struggling silently with crushing misery, so few get help. There are 100,000 Eleanors in this country who haven't been correctly diagnosed and who aren't receiving treatment that could mean the difference between life and death.

Even today, too many Americans are intolerant of any type of mental illness—*especially* depression, which is often dismissed as some sort of moral failure. In a recent poll by the National Institute of Mental Health, nearly half of all respondents stated that depression was a "personal weakness"—certainly not a health problem.

It was precisely this intolerance that drove a noted Pennsylvania jurist to try to cover up his depression by having his employees fill his Prozac prescriptions—a felony for which he will probably pay with his job. He finally confessed to the subterfuge because he said he decided that worse than being branded "depressed" was being labeled a drug trafficker.

Depression reaches from the poorest inner-city homes to the loftiest palaces. Sylvia Plath, Dick Cavett, Georgia O'Keeffe, Mark Twain, Virginia Woolf, and Abraham Lincoln all wrestled with depression.

"I felt a kind of numbness, an enervation," recalls William Styron in his book *Darkness Visible: A Memoir of Madness,* an account of his herculean struggle with major depression. "Mysteriously and in ways that are totally remote from normal experience, the gray drizzle of horror induced by depression takes on the quality of physical pain."

Is It the Blues—or Depression?

Of course, we all feel a little sad, dejected, or blue now and then. Fleeting unhappiness may briefly cloud your horizon after you lose a job, break up with your lover, or move to a new town. The profound mourning following the death of a loved one may last for several months—a completely normal response to a deeply felt emotional loss. The key difference between sad feelings and a true major depression is that sad feelings eventually pass, according to Douglas Jacobs, a Harvard Medical School psychiatrist who has devised national screening programs for depression.

"There were lots of times when I felt blue or sad," notes Sarah, 42, a North Carolina secretary. "Even when my divorce came through and my father died three weeks later, I managed to work through my sad feelings. But when I experienced major depression, it was very different.

"Before that, I had no idea what true depression was all about," Sarah explains. "Now there is a big "D" and a little "d" for me. Whenever people say that depression isn't a real mental disease, I find myself explaining just how terrible it can be."

As Sarah discovered, major depression is far more persistent than simple sadness. It descends as a sort of psychic cloud, numbing the soul with the conviction that the bleak outlook *will never change*. It interferes with sleep, appetite, sexual interest, self-image, and attitude. If you suffer from major depression, you can't just "snap out of it." And these dreadful feelings can last for weeks, months, or even years.

It is a disorder that costs this country dearly. The federal government estimates the cost of all types of depression is $43.7 billion each year—$12.4 billion in medical, psychiatric, and drug costs; $7.5 billion in depression-related suicide; and $23.8 billion in work absenteeism and lost productivity.

While effective therapy for depression has been available for decades, the condition is seriously undertreated in the United States, according to a panel of mental health experts reporting in the February 1997 *Journal of the American Medical Association*. This could either be due to the fact that doctors don't have the necessary training to effectively treat depression or because they may not view the condition seriously enough.

"There is still an enormous gap between our knowledge about the correct diagnosis and treatment of depression and the actual treatment that is being received in this country, " wrote the panel led by psychiatrist Robert M.A. Hirschfield, M.D., at the University of Texas at Galveston.

Some studies have shown that only one in 10 Americans with depression get adequate treatment. When left untreated, depression can interfere with personal relationships and job performance and can increase your risk for other illnesses, according to a panel organized by the National Depressive and Manic Depressive Association. It's the fourth leading public health problem in the world, yet only one in every three suffering from depression ever seeks help.

Major depression can be very hard to recognize, because it's a chronic, progressive disease. If you have major depression, you may go into remission, but chances are that without treatment, it usually strikes again, more quickly and more powerfully than before.

Are You Depressed?

A diagnosis may begin with a brief family history combined with a medical workup, including tests to rule out underactive thyroid, mononucleosis, anemia, diabetes, adrenal insufficiency, and hepatitis. Your doctor will want to know about any medications you've been taking, since a number of prescription drugs can cause depression (see box: "Drugs That Can Cause Depression"). While you're at it, you might also let your doctor know about any vitamins, herbal medicines, amino acids, diet supplements, or recreational drugs you have taken.

ARE YOU DEPRESSED?

➤ Emotions: Do you feel ineffably sad or cry a great deal?

➤ Appetite/weight: Have you gained or lost weight? Do you binge or overeat?

➤ Sleep: Do you have chronic insomnia or excessive sleepiness? Are you tired all the time, regardless how much sleep you get?

➤ Anger: Do you experience outbursts of complaints or shouting? Have you been feeling resentful and angry?

➤ Outlook: Have you lost interest in hobbies or activities that you formerly enjoyed?

➤ Libido: Have you lost interest in sex?

➤ Self-esteem: Do you feel worthless, unattractive, inappropriately guilty?

➤ Concentration: Do you have a hard time concentrating? Are your thoughts muddy or foggy?

➤ Anxiety: Do you brood, have phobias, delusions or fears?

➤ Restlessness: Do you have trouble sitting still?

➤ Muted affect: Do you have slow body movements and speech?

➤ Suicide: Have you thought you'd be better off dead?

Major Depression

While symptoms differ from one person to the next, major depression is almost always characterized by general feelings of sadness and a total loss of pleasure in things that once brought you joy. You might also have sleep and eating problems or a sense of worthlessness. Perhaps you're no longer interested in sex, you're feeling apathetic, or you have suicidal thoughts.

According to the fourth edition of the *Diagnostic and Statistical Manual of Mental Disorders*, published by the American Psychiatric Association, a typical episode of a major depressive disorder lasts at least two weeks and includes most of the symptoms listed in the box, "Are You Depressed?"

Other common signs of depression may not be found in medical journals. "I ask patients if there are cobwebs in their house," says psychiatrist Andy Myerson, M.D. "If patients aren't bathing, if their house isn't clean, if they can't get out of bed—that's a good indication that they're depressed."

Many people in the midst of depression agree with him. "If I have to fight my way to the bathroom and I haven't opened my mail," Violet laughs, "I know I'm in trouble."

It is possible, however, to have a major depression and not feel particularly sorrowful, sad, or hurting. You may instead have eating problems or problems sleeping, remembering, concentrating, or making decisions. Only a mental health expert can diagnose a depression that is hiding as some of these symptoms.

Dysthymic Disorder

Not everyone gets depressed in the same way. If you have a major depression (known as unipolar or clinical depression), your feelings of misery may be interrupted by periods when you feel okay. On the other hand, if you have a chronic minor depression (now called "dysthymic disorder"), you'll feel mildly depressed all the time; this constant low-level depression can last for years at a stretch. You may even have both types of depression at the same time.

"My problem with dysthymic disorder was characterized by fatigue," says Aguri, a 45-year-old psychologist who lives in New York. "By the afternoon, I became very tired and less clear in my thinking; I had to take a nap every afternoon or I couldn't work in the evening." Burdened by mounting job responsibilities, he finally sought help from his physician, who suggested the tricyclic Elavil. "It really helps," Aguri reports. "When I lower the dose or stop taking it, I can't sleep well and I get very tired. It helps improve my energy level."

Called depressive neurosis in the 1950s and depressive personality in the 1970s, dysthymic disorder is a persistent mild type of depression affecting as many as 3 million people. In order to be diagnosed with dysthymic disorder, you must have been depressed during most of the past two years, with at least two of the following six symptoms:

> ➤ Low self-esteem

> ➤ Poor appetite or overeating

> ➤ Insomnia or increased sleeping

> ➤ Difficulty concentrating or making decisions

➤ Hopelessness

➤ Fatigue or low energy

This type of mild depression can be misdiagnosed as borderline personality disorder, which in itself does not respond to antidepressants. Dysthymic disorder, however, can be treated with antidepressants.

Double Depression

If you've been struggling with a long-term dysthymic disorder and suddenly experience a major depression, your psychiatrist will diagnose a "double depression." Many doctors have successfully used the new SSRIs, including Prozac, in such cases to treat the dysthymic disorder and prevent the return of major depression. Controlling this combination of depressions may require a slightly higher dosage.

Atypical Depression

If you find that you continually crave sleep, food, or sex over a period of two weeks or more, you may be developing what's called "atypical depression."

Most depressed people don't sleep or eat enough, and many lose weight, but people with atypical depression *gain* weight and sleep too much. They're also anxious and extremely sensitive to their environment and to rejection.

Atypical depressions may be disguised as bulimia, anorexia, compulsive overeating, oversleeping, addictions, or impulsiveness. While some of these symptoms are also found in major depression, they aren't as severe and don't last as long. If you have an atypical depression, you may feel that your phobias, symptoms, or hysterical feelings are more troublesome than your depression, but, in fact it's the depression that causes these symptoms.

Experts don't know why atypical depression appears in many ways as the polar opposite of major depression or why it's more common in women than men. But we do know that without treatment, the symptoms will probably get worse. In the past, patients like this responded best to one of the MAOIs; today, the SSRIs (including Prozac) appear to be just as effective.

Subclinical Depression

If you have only two or three symptoms of depression as opposed to five or more, your doctor may diagnose a "subclinical depression." If you're so diagnosed, it is likely that you've never sought mental health treatment, since you can probably function fairly well despite low self-confidence, timidity, lack of interest, sadness, emptiness, or fatigue. Psychotherapy alone may not solve these problems if they are of long standing, but many people with subclinical depression respond well to Prozac or another SSRI in conjunction with psychotherapy.

Other Forms of Depression

The symptoms of psychotic depression may include delusions of guilt, serious medical illness, and a feeling of deserving punishment for imagined mistakes. There may also be auditory hallucinations or other delusions. The melancholic type of depression includes lack of the ability to have even fleeting good feelings, a worsening of mood in the morning, early morning awakening (between three and four o'clock), more than 5-percent weight loss per month, agitation or lethargy, loss of interest in all activities.

Manic Depression (Bipolar Disorder)

A person with manic depression suffers through alternating periods of severe depression and manic "highs" that can be severe enough to require hospitalization. When you experience a manic phase, you may be elated, irritable, or paranoid—you're probably hyperactive, concentrating on all sorts of risky activities. During this phase, you might talk very quickly and loudly, switching from one topic to another. You might go for days without rest, spend money you don't have, become promiscuous, eat and drink too much, or begin to think you can conquer the world. You might entice others to join you in wild business schemes. Eventually, you may begin to have serious delusions about your own abilities.

But after days or weeks of feeling all-powerful, suddenly you come crashing to earth in a profound depression that leaves you feeling defeated and doomed. The world that just yesterday was bright and full of promise is today a bleak and gray disaster.

John was a successful pediatrician when he was diagnosed with manic depression in his early thirties. For some years, his behavior had become increasingly erratic; periods of wild enthusiasm would be followed by months of black despair during which he dragged himself through seemingly endless days and sleepless nights. During one manic phase, he became obsessed with a pyramid scheme for selling auto products. Soon his entire home was converted into a

warehouse, and he listened to motivational tapes produced by company executives at all hours of the day and
night. His obsession soon drove him to harangue patients
and colleagues to join him in selling the products or listening to the tapes. Not until both his practice and his
professional reputation were in serious jeopardy was he
induced to seek treatment.

Manic depression can strike anyone. Some of history's
most creative individuals are now believed to have been
manic depressives. Some even created masterpieces during
a manic phase.

Like other forms of depression, manic depression
appears to be caused by a biochemical imbalance in the
brain that requires a combined treatment of medications
(including lithium) and therapy. While there is strong evidence that manic depression has a genetic component,
just because a sister, brother or parent has the disease
doesn't mean you're doomed to follow the same path. In
many cases, too much stress trips a biological vulnerability
mechanism and pushes a person into manic depression.

Suicide Risk

Because the primary risk of depression is suicide, a good
diagnosis and effective treatment are critical. At least 80
percent of suicides never got that treatment (see box:
"Warning Signs of Potential Suicide"). Even more frightening, suicide is the eighth leading cause of death in this
country—and the second leading cause of death among
teenagers. It's estimated that 30,000 Americans kill themselves each year, and at least 10 times that number make
unsuccessful attempts. The problem is particularly troubling

among the young: five teenagers a day commit suicide in
the United States. Although the rate among adolescents
tripled from 1957 to 1987, it stabilized in the late 1980s.
For every teenager who commits suicide, about 200 try.
Moreover, research shows that those who have ever

WARNING SIGNS OF POTENTIAL SUICIDE

A person thinking about suicide may show one or
more of the following symptoms, but these are
only guidelines. There is no single "typical" suicide
profile. A person showing suicidal signs should be
encouraged to seek professional help as soon as
possible. Start by calling local suicide hotlines or
a local psychiatrist or psychologist immediately.

➤ Suicide threats—The widespread belief that
  people who threaten suicide never follow
  through on that threat is not true.
➤ Withdrawal—an overwhelming urge to be
  alone or an unwillingness to communicate,
  withdrawing into a shell. Trouble with grades
  or on the job can signal such a retreat.
➤ Life crisis—Death, divorce, job loss, or accident
  can trigger suicide in a deeply depressed person.
➤ Behavior change—changes in appearance,
  energy, or attitude.
➤ Aggression—sudden interest in dangerous pur-
  suits, sports, or unsafe sexual practices.
➤ Moodiness— Sudden calm after severe depression may indicate a person has chosen suicide
  as a solution to problems.
➤ Gift-giving—sudden bequeathing of treasured
  possessions.

been hospitalized for depression have a 15 percent higher risk for suicide.

While suicide is more common among men, women make four times as many attempts. It's most prevalent among the elderly, those without a significant partner in their lives, with chronic medical problems and those with mood disorders.

Most people who are seriously depressed admit to having suicidal thoughts at some point, and many act on those thoughts.

Causes of Depression

The majority of experts agree that depression has no one specific cause. Instead, it's the result of a collision between genetics, biochemistry, and psychological factors.

Neurotransmitters

The physiological basis of depression can be found in nerve cells in the part of the brain responsible for human emotions centered in the hypothalamus, a cherry-size structure that controls basic functions such as thirst, hunger, sleep, sexual desire, and body temperature. Each nerve cell in your brain is separated by tiny gaps; neurotransmitters communicate by ferrying messages across these gaps to a "receptor" on the other side. Each neurotransmitter has a special shape that helps it fit exactly into a corresponding receptor like a key in an ignition switch. When the neurotransmitter "key" is inserted into its matching receptor's "ignition," the cell fires and sends the message on its way. Once the message is sent, the neurotransmitter is either absorbed into the cell or burned up by enzymes patrolling the gaps.

When the levels of these neurotransmitters are abnormally low, messages can't get across the gaps, and communication in the brain slows down. It appears that depression occurs if you don't have enough of these neurotransmitters circulating in your brain or if your neurotransmitters can't fit into the receptors for some reason.

While there are as many as 100 different kinds of neurotransmitters, norepinephrine, serotonin, and dopamine seem to be of particular importance in depression. The pathways for these neurotransmitters reach deep into many of the parts of the brain responsible for functions that are affected in depression—sleep, appetite, mood, and sexual interest.

Scientists aren't sure whether depression is directly related to abnormal levels of these transmitters, or whether these neurotransmitters affect yet another neurotransmitter that's even more directly involved in depression. But it is clear that neurotransmitters are related to depression because medications that boost levels of these neurotransmitters also ease depression. Yet some of the newer antidepressants don't affect the levels of all of these neurotransmitters, though they still relieve depression. And other drugs (such as cocaine) that *do* interfere with neurotransmitter levels *don't* affect depression.

And here's the knottiest puzzle of all: Antidepressants can raise your neurotransmitter levels almost immediately, but your depression won't lift until weeks after drug therapy has begun. Depression appears to be far more than a simple problem with the amount of neurotransmitters in the synaptic cleft. Instead, it is probably influenced by a complex interplay of receptor "ignition" responses and the release of the neurotransmitter "keys." It also seems to depend not just on the *number* of neurotransmitter keys but on the *quality* and *availability* of the receptor ignitions.

Antidepressants appear to make certain receptors unreachable, which may explain the antidepressants' lag time. The inaccessibility of these receptors may trigger an increase in the production of neurotransmitters. These changes don't happen right after antidepressant treatment begins; they can take up to several weeks. This receptor change has been reported in almost all antidepressant drug treatment and also in electroconvulsive therapy.

Loss and Trauma

Most cases of depression seem to be triggered by a serious loss or unpleasant experience that pushes a person who may be genetically or psychologically susceptible into a depressive abyss.

That's what happened to Rod, 31, when his mother—his last surviving relative—suddenly died. Rod came from a troubled family dogged by alcoholism and depression. When his long-suffering mother finally succumbed to a heart attack, Rod's world fell apart, and he entered a downward spiral of ever-deepening depression.

"Everything seemed gray and muffled," he recalled, "as if it were wrapped in cotton wool. Nothing had any color. Food had no taste. I couldn't sleep at night, and I'd stumble through my work."

In a study of 680 pairs of female twins, recent stress (a divorce, illness, bereavement, or legal problem) was the best predictor of depression. Other studies have found that as many as 86 percent of major depressions were set off by a life crisis.

At other times, a depressive disorder may seem to come out of the blue. It may be triggered by a physical illness, or it could be associated with hormonal changes after childbirth or during menopause. Some people become depressed after taking certain drugs (such as birth-control pills, steroids, or sleeping pills).

That was the case with Cathy, whose serious manic depression was triggered by massive doses of prednisone following a transplant operation.

"I was overdosed on prednisone," she reports, "and it made me feel terrible. I was a zombie."

Hormones

For some time, scientists have noticed that depression and problems with hormone regulation appear to go hand in hand. This link isn't really surprising, since hormones affect neurotransmitter activity, and neurotransmitters affect the timing and release of hormones. You may have noticed that depression tends to crop up during events related to reproduction (menstruation, ovulation, pregnancy, and menopause). Altered hormone levels during these times can affect mood-regulating neurotransmitters, but just how they accomplish this isn't clear.

PMS and Depression

Premenstrual syndrome (PMS) is usually associated with depression, irritability, exhaustion, sore breasts, bloating, and crying spells and affects most women in their twenties and thirties. Between 20 and 80 percent of women have some form of this problem, but according to the American Psychological Association Task Force on Women and Depression, only 5 percent experience significant discomfort and need professional treatment.

"I didn't have to look at a calendar to know when my period was due," confessed Kathy, 33, who suffers from premenstrual syndrome. "I'd start getting cranky and irritable a few days before my period, and then I'd get depressed. I'd snap at my family, and some days I just stayed in bed because I couldn't face the world. Then as soon as my period was over, I'd be perky as ever."

A woman's menstrual cycle is regulated by complex interactions between neurotransmitters (serotonin, dopamine, and norepinephrine), pituitary hormones, and ovarian hormones. We don't yet know exactly how the ovarian hormones interact with neurotransmitters or why the result varies so widely from one woman to the next, but it may have something to do with genetics. Your brain's ability to regulate neurotransmitters is strongly influenced by heredity.

Recent research at the University of California at San Diego found that some women who are depressed as a result of PMS have lower amounts of a brain chemical called melatonin when they sleep. Melatonin is released by the pineal gland to induce sleep and regulate circadian rhythms. Experts believe melatonin may suppress mood and mental quickness.

In fact, recent research has isolated serotonin as a possible culprit in PMS. In the late 1980s, several studies revealed that women who had PMS had lower serotonin levels right before their periods than women who don't have PMS.

There may also be a link between serotonin levels, carbohydrate cravings, and PMS, according to similar studies at the Massachusetts Institute of Technology by neuroscientist Richard Wurtman and Judith Wurtman, a cell biologist and nutritionist. They have found that depression, carbohydrate craving, and a few other PMS symptoms can be relieved by the drug D-fenfluramine, which affects serotonin.

If you experience one week during the month when you don't feel normal, you may be diagnosed as having PMS; if your negative emotions occur all month long but are aggravated premenstrually, your problem might more correctly be diagnosed as a mood disorder.

While there are no well-established treatments that work consistently for PMS, many doctors are now using antidepressants to treat severe cases; both Prozac and the tricyclic nortriptyline have been reported to be of particular benefit to women with severe symptoms. Lithium has also been used successfully in certain types of PMS.

"We use [Prozac] for a great number of women with PMS, and the results are wonderful," reports one psychiatric nurse, who is certified to treat patients in practice with a psychiatrist. "You'd be surprised at how well it works for all the symptoms of PMS."

Try keeping a daily rating scale for several months. It's the best way to establish a link between your mood and your periods.

Of course, it could also be true that many women have mild depressions that respond well to antidepressants; once their depression is treated, the PMS-like symptoms disappear.

It's also important to realize that some cases of PMS may actually be an undiagnosed depression. In one study, two-thirds of the women with a history of major depression experienced more symptoms of PMS than those who were not chronically depressed. *Even after menopause,* many of these women still experienced PMS symptoms even though they didn't have the hormonal fluctuations that had supposedly triggered their PMS. This suggests that for *some* women, what appears to be PMS may in fact be an untreated depression.

Postpartum Depression

Up to 70 percent of all new mothers experience the "baby blues," a mild form of brief depression including crying spells, restlessness, feelings of unreality and confusion, depersonalization, guilt, and negative feelings toward both the husband and the child. Symptoms often fade within a week.

While the symptoms are well documented, scientists aren't sure whether these feelings are simply the result of a profound life-role change or a true metabolic disruption. However, it's clear that five days after delivery, the levels of estrogen and progesterone drop, and a burst of pro-lactin occurs. The lower the progesterone falls, the more likely it is that the mother will become depressed within 10 days after birth.

"I'd read about the baby blues, but I didn't really expect to feel sad," recalls Wanda, who had her first child at age 36. "I was always so perky. I've never been depressed in my life. But when I heard them wheeling my baby down the corridor to my room, my heart would actually sink. I felt terrible that instead of being thrilled at the prospect of seeing my baby, I just wanted to be left alone.

I would lie in bed, and tears would roll down my cheeks for no apparent reason."

For Wanda, these feelings faded within a day or two. Other women aren't so lucky. One or two out of every ten new mothers struggle with a more serious form of depression, which may last from six weeks to a year or more. These women worry constantly about their child's health and their own ability to have normal motherly feelings.

An even smaller number, just .01 percent to .02 percent, will develop postpartum psychosis between the third and fourteenth day after birth. This frightening development can appear quickly, ballooning from a moderate depression to delusions and hallucinations. In most cases, there is no prior history of depression and its occurrence seems to have nothing to do with other events in the woman's life. This high-risk condition must be treated with hospitalization, medication, and sometimes electro-shock therapy.

In general, women with a history of depression or manic depression before pregnancy are at higher risk for developing postpartum depression.

Endocrine Disorders

There are several hormonal or endocrine diseases that may cause depression, including hypothyroidism (underactive thyroid gland), hyperthyroidism (overactive thyroid gland), Addison's disease (underactive adrenal gland), Cushing's syndrome (overactive adrenal gland) and either under-or-overactivity of the parathyroid gland. Hormonal drugs (including birth-control pills and steroids like cortisone and prednisone) may also cause depression.

Puberty

Puberty is the first of a series of reproduction-related events that appear to be strongly linked with depression. One study found that a woman's first major depressive episode was most likely to occur around the age of 13 or 14. A study of 1,500 New York youngsters found that severe depression affects 7 percent of all girls. But it's not just young women who suffer with depression at this age. Boys, too, can experience hormonal changes together with the problems of emerging identity, peer pressure, sexual issues, and increasing adult responsibilities, all combining to cause depression during adolescence.

Menopause and Depression

The idea that menopause and depression are interrelated phenomena is a hot potato widely disputed by many feminists. It's a fact that women go through hormonal changes during menopause, but scientists have been able to prove no clear-cut relationship between depression and menopause. Some experts believe that you may experience mood changes once your estrogen levels drop. Others suggest that low thyroid levels that often occur at this time may also influence depression.

The reduction of estrogen following menopause causes several problems, including osteoporosis (thinning of the bones), dryness and thinning of the vaginal walls, and an increased risk of heart disease. According to Dr. Ellen McGrath, chair of the American Psychological Association National Task Force on Women and Depression, women are probably more likely to be depressed over these physical changes than over the ending of menstruation.

Heart Disease and Depression

People who are depressed are more than twice as likely than others to develop high blood pressure, a major cause of heart disease, according to a study by the National Center for Health Statistics of the Centers for Disease Control and Prevention in Atlanta. Even intermediate levels of anxiety and depression were associated with a 60 percent greater likelihood of developing high blood pressure. While the link between depression and heart disease is found in both black and white patients, the risk is especially high for blacks.

Moreover, depressed people are four times more likely to have a heart attack than those with more positive states of mind, according to a study at the Johns Hopkins School of Hygiene and Public Health. In addition, people who are depressed are more likely to smoke, which is another known cause of heart disease.

Those with the highest levels of depression and anxiety were at greatest risk of developing high blood pressure. But even those with intermediate levels of anxiety and depression were also associated with hypertension.

Scientists suggest that the link between depression and heart disease may be due to biochemical changes that occur in depressed people, such as the secretion of stress hormones that weaken the immune system. Others believe depression leaves victims so unhappy that they neglect their health, forget to take medications like those that control high blood pressure, and thus become more vulnerable to heart attacks.

Migraines

The severe headache known as migraine, with accompanying symptoms of nausea, diarrhea and visual disturbances, attacks about 8 million Americans, 75 percent of them women. They are believed to be linked to changes in the levels of estrogen and serotonin. Depression and stress also contribute to migraines.

Because of the suspected role of serotonin in migraine attacks, some doctors have been successful in treating them with a standard dose of one of the new SSRIs—Prozac, Zoloft or Paxil—which act exclusively on the serotonin system.

Heredity

Although there's no certain evidence that there is a single gene for depression, some families have an inherited vulnerability to depression. This is especially true in the case of manic depression, where up to 50 percent of manic-depressives have at least one parent with the disorder.

"My father was an alcoholic and my brother is a manic-depressive," notes Eleanor. "It's not surprising that I have a problem with depression, too."

Science would tend to agree with her. A 1992 study of female identical twins found that if one twin has a major depression, the other (who shares all her genes) is 66-percent more likely to suffer from the same problem than are unrelated children. But among fraternal female twins (who share no more genes than non-twin sisters), one twin had only a 27-percent higher chance of sharing the other's depression.

Researchers have concluded that a person may not inherit depression solely as a result of one gene, the way you inherit hair or eye color. At most, say experts at the Medical College of Virginia, depression is probably only about 40 percent influenced by genes. People *can* inherit certain personality traits, collectively known as "depressive personality disorder," that may make them prone to depression. People with the disorder tend to be pessimistic and brooding, with an overly critical attitude toward themselves and others. It's also true that if you're seriously depressed, you may have a different sort of biochemistry, with high levels of the stress chemical cortisol and low levels of the calming neurotransmitters serotonin and norepinephrine.

WHAT ARE YOUR CHANCES OF INHERITING DEPRESSION?

➤ Relatives: Close relatives of depressed people have a 15 percent chance of inheriting major depression.

➤ Twins: If your identical twin is depressed, you're 67 percent more likely to be depressed.

➤ Substance abuse: If your depressed relatives abuse alcohol or drugs as a symptom of depression, you're eight to ten times more likely to do the same.

➤ Suicide: If you become depressed, you're much more vulnerable to suicide a close relative has committed suicide.

➤ Women: Close female relatives of depressed women have a one in four chance of inheriting major depression and a 90-percent chance of having mild depression.

Biological Rhythms

Your body's internal rhythm waxes and wanes with the ticking of the clock. For example, your body temperature rises during the day and falls during the evening. Biological rhythms such as hormone secretion and sleep-wake patterns have a 24-hour cycle and are called circadian rhythms.

It's not surprising that there may be a link between depression and biological rhythms, too. You may find your moods get better or worse in tune with the seasons or the time of day. Perhaps you've noticed that you tend to feel terrible in the morning but a bit better as the day wears on. Or maybe you feel worse and worse as the day proceeds.

"I was always at my worst during the morning," says Jennifer, 42, who takes Effexor to manage her depression. "Now, from 8:30 A.M. to 11 A.M., I'm feeling the way I wanted to feel for the last 20 years. I'm not weighted down by an ungodly weight."

Early-morning awakening is one of the hallmarks of clinical depression, and the continuing cycles of depression and mania are the hallmarks of manic depression.

Seasonal Affective Disorder

The syndrome of winter depression, called seasonal affective disorder (SAD), is specifically related to changes in the length of daylight across the seasons. While its exact cause is unknown, the disorder has been linked to a malfunction in the body's biological clock that controls temperature and hormone production.

As many as 12 million Americans may suffer from this disorder, and up to 35 million others may experience milder forms. It's at least four times as common among women, usually beginning in the twenties and thirties (although it has been reported in some children and teenagers). Other estimates suggest that as many as half of all women in northern states experience pronounced winter depression, but very few receive the necessary treatment because their doctors don't know how to tell the difference between typical depressive symptoms and SAD.

"I start to feel depressed around November," says Anne, 40, a Pennsylvania probation officer. "It just keeps

---

WHERE TO BUY LIGHT FIXTURES TO TREAT SEASONAL AFFECTIVE DISORDER

Light boxes for the treatment of SAD are usually metal with fluorescent bulbs inside. Some are full-spectrum (including a small among of ultraviolet light), and some aren't.

The Sunbox Company
19217 Orbit Drive
Gaithersburg, MD   20879
(800-LITE-YOU) (800-548-3968)

Apollo Light Systems, Inc.
352 West 1060 South
Orem, UT   84058
(800-545-9667)

Hughes Lighting Technologies
Yacht Club Drive
Lake Hopatcong, NJ   07849
(201-663-1214)

getting worse until the spring. It helps a little bit if I take naps, but what I really seem to need is the sunlight."

The pineal gland appears to be particularly important in the development of SAD. Nestling near the center of the brain, the gland processes information about light through special nerve pathways and releases the sleep-inducing hormone melatonin, also responsible for regulating circadian rhythms. Melatonin is produced in the dark and peaks during the winter. Experts believe it may suppress mood and mental quickness. Interestingly, manic-depressives are extremely sensitive to light, and exposure to it causes their melatonin levels to plummet.

Your body is regulated by some sort of biological clock that sets the pace for everyday rhythms of sleep, activity, temperature, and cortisol and melatonin release. Most people maintain a certain flexibility in this system, allowing them to synchronize this biological clock to environmental changes. But experts suspect that some people—perhaps those prone to depression—don't synchronize their clocks so easily. It could be that their internal clock is out of step with the world's 24-hour rhythm, so that melatonin is released too early (causing evening sleepiness and early-morning awakening) or too late (causing insomnia and trouble waking up).

In some cases, SAD eventually disappears, but in others it persists for a lifetime. The best treatment for this disorder is phototherapy—exposure to special types of light during the winter—which will reverse this type of depression in most people.

Animal research suggests that light therapy eases depression by helping to boost serotonin levels.

Researchers found that when hamsters were subjected to pulses of light, the levels of available serotonin in their brains rose. These findings, published in the January 1997 issue of *Nature*, also suggest that light therapy might help those with other disorders associated with low serotonin levels, such as obsessive-compulsive disorder.

SAD can be effectively and inexpensively treated, but you must be sure to get an accurate diagnosis and the right kind of light box to provide enough high-intensity light for a certain time each day. After a few days of your sitting for several hours under special fluorescent lights, symptoms subside; they reappear if treatment stops. In general, patients must sit about three feet away from a bank of special lights of between six and eight fluorescent bulbs about three hours daily (for suppliers of these bulbs, see box). Homemade versions can also be built. Ordinary room light is not bright enough to affect SAD.

While researchers are still studying this treatment, many physicians recommend it for this type of depression. *Treatment should be under the supervision of an expert.* Experts believe that the treatment works by increasing the secretion of melatonin in the brain, helping to regulate your circadian rhythms.

Because light therapy may be only partly successful in eradicating symptoms, treatment may be bolstered by the use of antidepressants. Antidepressants may be used alone instead of light therapy for people with SAD, but the two treatments are usually combined, which often means that lower doses of antidepressants are needed.

Don't be surprised if your doctor must adjust the dose of antidepressants with the changing seasons, increasing your dose as the days become shorter, decreasing it as the days lengthen.

More and more doctors are considering Prozac and the other SSRIs to be the drugs of choice for SAD, primarily because the serotonin system is believed to be part of the problem in this disorder. Desyrel has also been used successfully with SAD patients. Older antidepressants may also be beneficial, such as the tricyclics desipramine or imipramine. (Doctors often stay away from the more sedating tricyclics, such as amitriptyline and doxepin, since people with SAD tend to sleep too much as it is.)

A few depressed people with problems in their basic circadian rhythm appear to be helped—at least temporarily—by staying up all night then resuming their regular sleep-wake cycle, but others don't get any benefit from this treatment at all. While experts aren't sure why this works, they think it has something to do with shifting the basic circadian rhythm back to a normal 24-hour cycle. However, this treatment is experimental and should not be attempted by the patient without consultation with a physician.

Drugs That Cause Depression

A number of drugs now on the market may actually *cause* depression (see box: "Drugs That Can Cause Depression"). These include blood-pressure medications such as Catapres, Aldomet, and Inderal; drugs used to treat Parkinson's disease such as L-dopa and bromocriptine; diet pills and medicines prescribed for arthritis, ulcers, or seizures; and hormones like estrogen, progesterone, cortisol, and prednisone.

Moreover, some commonly prescribed tranquilizers such as Valium or Halcion, which are designed to calm you down, can on rare occasions stimulate violence, aggression, or depression. Styron described just such an occurrence in *Darkness Visible*. Because he suffered from insomnia as a result of his severe depression, he was given the sleeping pill Halcion. When he took inappropriately excessive doses, his depression appeared to get much worse. Styron blames the drug as a contributory factor in his downward spiral into profound depression.

DRUGS THAT CAUSE DEPRESSION

Drug-induced depression is more likely to be found in those who are genetically vulnerable to this disorder. The following drugs are known to cause depression in some people:

> Benzodiazepines
> Clonidine
> Cortisone-like steroids
> Digitalis
> Indomethacin
> Levodopa
> Methyldopa
> Oral contraceptives
> Phenothiazines (some)
> Reserpine

Who Gets Depressed?

About 3 percent to 4 percent of Americans experience major depression. About 5 percent of Americans struggle with other forms of depression—dysthymic disorder (mild depression), chronic treatment-resistant depression, or depression caused by medical or other psychiatric disorders. Manic depression affects another 1 to 2 percent.

If you've had one episode of major depression, you've got a 50-percent chance of having another bout—sometimes four or five episodes during a lifetime. Some people have recurrent depressive episodes separated by years of relatively good mental health. Others experience clusters of depression over a short period with a few glimpses of normal function in between. Unfortunately, as many as 35 percent of depressed people experience a chronic form of the condition that never fades away at all without treatment.

The problem appears to be on the increase. In this century, each succeeding generation has experienced major depressions at earlier and earlier ages, and each generation that follows the next has a higher lifetime risk of experiencing the disorder.

Women and Depression

More than twice as many women as men are diagnosed with depression, although the reason why this occurs is still hotly debated. Today, experts predict that one in four women will experience a depressive episode sometime during her life. Some experts blame physiology—heredity or hormonal imbalances. Others point to the different ways men and women learn to handle emotions, and the fact that health professionals more readily diagnose depression in women. Some blame social factors: a woman's lower economic status and susceptibility to abuse contribute to higher rates of depression. Physical and sexual abuse may also be major factors in women's depression, according to psychologist Ellen McGrath, author of *When Feeling Bad Is Good*. Experts have estimated that between 37 percent and 50 percent of women have had a significant experience of physical or sexual abuse before age 21. For many women, McGrath believes, depression may actually be the effects of post-traumatic stress syndrome.

Careful epidemiological studies have shown that the higher depressive ratio for women is *not* due to a woman's greater willingness to report depressive episodes, women really *do* get depressed at a higher rate.

The typical depressed woman is between 25 and 40, married, and raising children. Research does suggest that depression is most likely to be found at both ends of the economic spectrum—in professional women and those with low income, as well as in those with little personal support and substance abusers.

What many have trouble accepting is that some of a woman's vulnerability to depression may be biological. In fact, one out of every ten women becomes seriously depressed after giving birth. Almost 90 percent report PMS symptoms, although they may not all be disturbed enough to qualify for a diagnosis of PMS. In women with PMS depression, serotonin levels are below those of women without PMS, and lower before their periods than afterward.

Depression in Childhood

Most children will get a bit sad now and then when something goes wrong at home or school. When youngsters get the blues, their sad feelings should pass within a few days. If the depression deepens or continues longer than two weeks, it could indicate a more serious problem.

While most people think of depression as a disorder of adulthood, in fact it can appear at any age—even in infancy. Depressed children may become clingy, tired, listless, or anxious. They may refuse to go to school and may try to hurt themselves (banging their head against a wall, for example). They may lose interest in normal activities and start having problems in school. If the child's depression is severe enough, even a youngster no more than five or six may deliberately attempt suicide.

"I didn't want to live anymore," whispered one-five-year-old boy as he lay dying after darting in front of a truck because he said he felt unloved.

A 1982 study of 3,000 children found that almost 15 percent of them had symptoms of depression; the same study found that by age 15, one out of five children depressed.

The average length of depression in childhood is about seven months, but the younger the child, the more serious the prognosis. Odds are great that a child who has experienced one major depression will have another episode.

If you take your child to the doctor because of your concern about depression, the doctor will probably first take a complete medical history, focusing on the child's feelings, psychological traits, and social background. The visit should include a thorough physical exam to rule out underlying physical disorders.

In recent years, more and more doctors have begun to realize that youngsters can suffer from a wide variety of mood disorders and that they can be just as sick as any adult. As a result, the use of antidepressants and lithium in childhood has become much more common.

Indeed medication may be an effective part of the treatment for several psychiatric disorders in childhood and adolescence, according to the American Academy of Child and Adolescent Psychiatry. If your doctor recommends medication for your child, he or she should be experienced in the treatment of psychiatric illnesses and should fully explain the reasons for the recommended drug, its benefits, side effects, and alternatives.

Parents must realize that medication should not be used alone but as part of a comprehensive treatment plan that usually includes some type of psychotherapy. In addition, your doctor should provide ongoing evaluation. When prescribed appropriately by an experienced psychiatrist, medication may help children and teenagers with psychiatric disorders feel better.

Psychiatric medication may be prescribed for a number of problems, including:

➤ *Depression*—lasting feelings of sadness, helplessness, hopelessness, unworthiness and guilt, inability to feel pleasure, declining school work, changes in sleeping or eating)

➤ *Eating disorder*—either anorexia nervosa or bulimia or a combination of the two

➤ *Manic depression* (bipolar disorder)— periods of depression alternating with manic periods, including

    irritability, happy moods, excessive energy, behavior
    problems, staying up late at night, and grand plans

When a child is diagnosed with a full-blown major depression, an antidepressant such as imipramine may be considered in order to bring the child out of the depression, thereby avoiding harming the child's emotional growth and relationships.

Most experts think that children who have one episode of depression early in life are at risk for future episodes. Some studies have found that as many as 10 percent of children who have been hospitalized for a suicide attempt will make a successful attempt within the next five years.

The use of antidepressants in children and adolescents is not without controversy, however, according to Theodore Petti, M.D., child and adolescent psychiatrist at Indiana University. While double-blind placebo-controlled studies of hospitalized children have not found much difference in effectiveness between tricyclic antidepressants and placebos, psychiatrists in actual practice *have* found that tricyclics can help ease a child's depression.

The tricyclics are generally the first-choice antidepressants for youngsters because doctors have so much long-term experience with them. "If I see a youngster for a couple of sessions and he doesn't appear to be responding to psychotherapy and he's really hampered in ordinary developmental tasks (such as schoolwork or family relationships), then I will seriously consider using an antidepressant," said Dr. Petti.

While the new SSRIs carry less risk of side effects, there have been no controlled studies among this age group. The major concern that doctors have with using tricyclics in children is the risk of death, presumably from heart problems, that has been associated with the tricyclic desipramine among hyperactive youngsters.

Depression in Adolescence

The picture of depression changes as the child enters adolescence. Many people experience their first bout with major depression during adolescence, although they may not know it. It commonly appears for the first time between ages 15 and 19; recent surveys reveal that as many as 20 percent of high-school students are deeply unhappy or have some kind of psychiatric problem. Suicide is a particular danger for this age group (see box: "Risk Factors for Teenage Suicide").

Depressed teenagers nearly always experience changes in thinking, such as low self-esteem and self-criticism. In this age group, depression is often disguised as substance abuse. It may be acted out in risk-taking or problems with authority. Depressed teenagers may become antisocial, restless, negative, oversensitive, uncooperative, or aggressive; they may abuse drugs or alcohol and stop going to school. Because most of these symptoms are to some degree considered typical of adolescent behavior in our culture, teenage depression often goes undiagnosed and untreated. This was what happened to Beth.

An 18-year-old athlete who had battled depression and weight problems for most of her teenage years, Beth always blamed her depression on her excess weight, but after shedding 75 pounds, she still felt smothered by a cloak of sadness. She became so despondent that her

Risk Factors for Teenage Suicide

➤ Previous attempts. Youths who attempt suicide remain vulnerable for several years, especially for the first three months following an attempt.

➤ Psychiatric history. Studies have shown that inpatient psychiatric care is associated with far more suicide attempts.

➤ Personal failure. High standards (the teen's or the parents') that are not met, even after only one setback, may set off a downward spiral ending in suicide.

➤ Recent loss. Death of close friends or family, divorce, or a breakup with a boyfriend or girlfriend may leave a teenager so lost and alone that suicide seems the only option.

➤ Substance abuse. Some teens abuse drugs or alcohol to self-medicate overwhelming depression; a combination of depression, substance abuse, and lowered impulse control can end in a suicide attempt.

➤ Family handguns. A gun in the house may make it easy for a troubled teen to commit suicide; children of law-enforcement officers have a much higher rate of suicide because of the accessibility of guns.

➤ Family violence. Violence in the home teaches youths that the way to resolve conflict is through violence.

➤ Communication lack. The inability to discuss angry or uncomfortable feelings within the family can lead to suicide.

weight loss had not made her happy that she was driven to hang herself in a tree near her home.

"Even after she lost all that weight," one of her friends recalled, "she smiled with her mouth, but never with her eyes."

Should a teenager you know be thinking of suicide, try to talk about these feelings immediately. Bringing up the subject won't plant ideas that weren't there, but it may help lessen feelings of isolation and entrapment. Ignoring suicidal thoughts or behavior will make suicide more likely to occur.

Depression in the Elderly

While older people also suffer from major depression, their condition is often misinterpreted or ignored. Experts estimate that up to 20 percent of the more than 30 million people over age 65 in this country may be experiencing a major depression. In fact, depression is more than four times more common in this age group than in the general population, and the suicide rate for people over 65 is fifteen times higher.

Depression is *not* a normal part of aging, although it's widely assumed to be, since old age in this country is so often associated with deprivation and loss. In fact, older people are no more "entitled" to feelings of misery than the rest of us.

Because depression in the later years can cause distractibility, indifference, memory problems, and disorientation, the condition is often misdiagnosed as senility. About 12 percent of elderly people who are diagnosed with dementia are really depressed. (It's also possible to be both demented *and* depressed.)

Moreover, many of the diseases that elderly people tend to get may appear as depression. These include Cushing's or Parkinson's disease, thyroid diseases, pulmonary disorders, vitamin deficiencies, cancer, and stroke. Inappropriate sedating drug treatment in nursing-home populations can also cause depression.

If you've been having some personality or mood changes, a doctor should give you a range of tests, including a CAT scan of the brain, blood tests (including thyroid-function tests), and perhaps an electroencephalogram. If these tests don't identify an underlying medical cause for your mood changes, there's a good chance that you may be depressed. If you or members of your family have ever been depressed before, this diagnosis is even more likely.

Because metabolism slows with age, elderly people often respond to smaller doses of antidepressants than younger people.

Treating Depression

As many as 90 percent of people with depression can be successfully treated, usually within 12 to 14 weeks.

One of the first tasks is to choose a mental health professional to diagnose and treat your depression—this could be a psychiatrist, nurse-psychotherapist, social worker, or family therapist. Some people choose a psychotherapist to assist them in understanding and dealing with their problems, and have a psychiatrist or general practitioner prescribe antidepressants and monitor their medical progress.

A psychiatrist has medical training and can prescribe drugs; other mental health professionals have psychotherapy training but can't prescribe medications. In many states, a nurse-psychotherapist may be licensed to prescribe medications in collaboration with a physician.

Of course, what's most important in whomever you choose is that you have trust and confidence in your therapist.

Psychotherapy

Many studies have suggested that the best results can be obtained from a combination of antidepressants and some type of psychotherapy. Even though depression is so responsive to a wide number of drugs, that doesn't mean it's not important to sit down and talk with your doctor to see what the depression is all about.

"Talk therapy" is probably most useful if your personality and life experiences are the primary cause of your depression. There are a number of different approaches.

Cognitive therapy is based on the idea that depression is a distortion in thinking, that how you feel is a direct product of how you think. Developed specifically to treat depression and anxiety by psychiatrist Aaron T. Beck, M.D., at the University of Pennsylvania, this type of therapy can pinpoint problem patterns of thinking that can result in depressive attitudes.

You'd be surprised how many people—without ever realizing what they're doing—develop a negative pattern of thinking that can automatically lead to depressed feelings. This negative personal outlook can become such a habit that it begins to interfere with everyday functioning.

If you have this problem, you may think that you've caused something to happen that in fact you're not responsible for ("personalization"), or you may exhibit an "all-or-nothing" attitude—believing that unless you're perfect, you've failed. Another typical distortion is "magnification" or "minimization," in which you blow up the importance of some things and discount the value of others.

If you see yourself in this pattern, cognitive therapy can help you understand more about your thought patterns and how to substitute positive thinking. You'll learn how to recognize and label these distortions and understand when you're using them.

Behavioral therapy is similar to cognitive therapy in that it teaches clients how to alter thought distortions, but it also seeks to alter behavior. Based on the idea that a depressed person isn't getting enough positive feedback, this type of therapy offers practical suggestions on how to reinforce healthy behavior via a system of self-rewards. This type of therapy is especially helpful if you have phobias or panic attacks.

Interpersonal therapy focuses on the development and improvement of relationships. Developed by psychiatrist Gerald Klerman, M.D., of Harvard University, and psychologist Myrna Weissman, Ph.D., of Yale University, this type of therapy helps people identify and resolve their problems with others. The client is helped to understand how important positive relationships are to mental health, to assess and define current relationships, and develop treatment goals. The client is taught relationship skills, focusing on the present instead of the past. Normally considered to be a short-term approach, it doesn't work for everyone. But for appropriate cases it can be very effective; a 1989 study by the National Institute of Mental Health found that 57 percent to 69 percent of clients who completed a 16-week course of interpersonal therapy no longer reported depressive symptoms and were more effective at work and at home.

Psychodynamic therapy, much like classical psycho-analysis, explores the past for the seeds of unresolved emotional conflict with a therapist who actively directs the therapy and offers suggestions and interpretations.

You may also benefit from *group therapy,* learning with other people about how best to cope with your depression. Groups can provide a source of connection that helps depressed people interact with others, build new relationships, and benefit from the feedback of others who have been in the same situation. Twelve-step self-help groups can be very helpful, since many people are depressed in part because of unresolved addictions. Because an addiction may interfere with depression recovery, participation in such self-help groups may help resolve depression.

But psychotherapy and antidepressants aren't the only ways to deal with depression.

Exercise

There's now solid evidence that regular aerobic exercise (such as running, biking, or swimming) can ease some more moderate cases of depression by raising the level of certain brain chemicals responsible for mood—some of the same brain chemicals that are affected by antidepressants. Even a brisk midday walk for 10 to 20 minutes can help. To be most effective, you should exercise regularly at least three times a week (five or more is better) for at least half an hour each time.

Don't expect to set Olympic records when you start out, however, or you'll be bound to get discouraged and quit. A combination of walking and running is a good way to start, since it's cheap (no equipment necessary) and you can do it either alone or in a group.

Exercise has not been shown to be effective for severe depression.

Electroshock Treatment

Despite its frightening reputation, electroconvulsive treatment (ECT), formerly known as shock therapy, may work for those very serious depressions that just don't respond to any other treatment, especially when there's a risk of suicide. The modern version of ECT is nothing like the sort of mental torture depicted in movies like *One Flew Over the Cuckoo's Nest*.

While many people believe that the origins of ECT lie in the ancient Roman tradition of applying electric eels to the head as a cure for madness, the true beginning of ECT occurred during the late 1700s. A machine using weak electric currents was used in Middlesex Hospital in England in 1767 to treat a range of illnesses; London brain surgeon John Birch used this machine to shock the brain of depressed patients. At about the same time, Benjamin Franklin was shocked into unconsciousness (and experienced brief memory loss) during one of his electricity experiments. He is said to have recommended electric shock for the treatment of mental illness.

The modern practice of electric shock treatment for the alleviation of depression and mental illness is less than 65 years old. It was a Hungarian psychiatrist who noticed a number of studies reporting that schizophrenia and epilepsy didn't occur in the same patient; he wondered if an artificially induced seizure might cure schizophrenia.

He began inducing seizures with camphor and other drugs, but Italian psychiatrist Ugo Cerletti and his colleagues explored the possibility of using electric shock to achieve similar results. Cerletti's version was considered an improvement over the drug-induced seizures, which were associated with toxic side effects.

Because it was cheap and easy, the use of ECT soon spread; by the 1950s it was the primary method of treatment for depression until the discovery of antidepressants led to a substantial decline in use.

How ECT Works

In modern ECT treatments, the patient is given an anesthetic and a muscle relaxant before padded electrodes are applied to one or both of the temples. A controlled electric pulse is delivered to the electrodes until the patient experiences a brain seizure; treatment usually consists of six to twelve seizures (two or three a week).

After the treatment, the patient may experience a period of confusion which is later forgotten, and a brief period of amnesia covering the period of time right before the treatment.

On regaining consciousness, patients who have received ECT seem much like those who have experienced post-traumatic amnesia. Tests on memory have revealed a temporary memory impairment; after a number of treatments some patients say they experience a more serious memory loss involving everyday forgetfulness, which usually disappears a few weeks after treatment. New research suggests that ECT given on only one side of the head produces equal benefit to the standard method without any accompanying memory loss.

The controversy surrounding ECT is likely to continue for some time, and it remains unclear whether ECT affects permanent memory. Many studies indicate that ECT doesn't have any extensive effect on permanent memory function. All patients show some amount of amnesia for events immediately before the treatment.

Some scientists believe that some people may falsely conclude their memory is impaired. In one study, scientists found significant differences between patients who report memory problems and those who don't. Those who complained tended to believe the ECT hadn't helped their depression, which could mean that their own assessment of memory might be the result of their continuing illness. Three years after treatment, this group insisted their amnesia remained, even though there was no objective proof of this. Researchers believe that their initial experience of true amnesia immediately after ECT might have caused them to question whether their memory function had ever recovered.

It is true, however, that ECT in older depressed people who are also demented can worsen their condition. It is also true that ECT can be abused as a treatment. Even ECT proponents admit there is a low incidence of adverse reaction to the treatment, although estimates of how great a risk vary.

ECT in Youth

While depressed teenagers are very much like depressed adults, psychiatrists rarely consider ECT for them, and there are no controlled studies for this age group. In a recent survey, 42 percent of child psychiatrists opposed ECT for young children and 19 percent opposed it for teenagers—even for adolescents with psychotic depression. On the other hand, 100 percent were willing to prescribe antidepressants.

The current attitude against ECT is based on a 1954 study of young schizophrenia patients treated with ECT seven years earlier, which found that benefits were temporary. Since then, 114 cases have been published in which results were said to be excellent. For example, a recent Mayo Clinic study of 20 teenagers found that ECT reduced or eliminated symptoms in those with manic depression and major depression. No adverse effects were reported.

While current research suggests that ECT doesn't harm intellectual development of children or adolescents, there is a risk of prolonged seizure, since youngsters have a greater susceptibility to seizures than adults. However, according to Max Fink, M.D., professor of psychiatry and neurology at SUNY/Stony Brook, prolonged seizures can be prevented by using less electrical energy, monitoring the duration of the seizure, and cutting the seizure short with an IV of anticonvulsant drugs, such as Valium.

According to Dr. Fink, teenage patients with severe depression or mania who don't respond to medication are often successfully treated with ECT. Too often, however, they are almost always given complex drug combinations that Dr. Fink believes may be more dangerous than ECT and not very effective. He believes that adolescents should be considered candidates for ECT in any situation where it would be appropriate for an adult.

Prepubescent children, however, are another matter. Because of the fear that repeated seizures might damage a maturing brain or interfere with development, it is not often considered to be a good treatment choice. ECT may be used successfully with a few such children suffering from overwhelming impulses to mutilate themselves and who have severe mental retardation.

Is ECT for You?

If your doctor is considering ECT for you, it's important to understand that this form of treatment doesn't combine very well with most antidepressants, including Prozac. As of 1993 there weren't any studies that showed any benefit of ECT and Prozac, and there have been rare cases of people on Prozac having prolonged seizures after ECT.

Since there doesn't seem to be a benefit in having people take antidepressants while receiving ECT, it's better to discontinue drug treatment three to ten days before ECT is scheduled. The only exception is in the case of suicidal patients, when there isn't time to wait until the drugs have left the system because their mood may be life-threatening. However, *after* ECT is given, antidepressants are usually prescribed to help maintain normal mood.

Conclusion

This chapter has presented a general overview of depression—what causes it, who's at risk, symptoms, and types of treatment. The next chapter will look at one specific type of treatment—antidepressants. You'll learn how these drugs were developed, their basic biochemical action, and how they might work for you.

2

ALL ABOUT ANTIDEPRESSANTS

---

*"When I was depressed, I was always overwhelmed.
It took me so long to do any normal job, just brushing
my teeth took forever. I felt doomed all the time. After
I took Effexor, I felt as if this terrible weight, this
slowing down, had been lifted."*

—Barbara, 49

There's no *best* way to treat all types of people and
depression. In fact, more and more psychiatrists are
coming to the conclusion that major recurrent depression
is a chronic disease that may require lifetime medication.
And while studies suggest that a combination of psychotherapy and antidepressants is the most effective
treatment for depression, for some chronically depressed
people talk therapy just doesn't help—and it can foster
deep feelings of resentment.

"I spent years in group therapy," says Jan, a 39-year-
old Boston nurse. "I spent decades talking to experts. I
came to realize that I'd put all the honesty a person could
muster into my therapy, and I still wasn't any better.
Something always felt *physically* wrong. I always felt I had

a biochemical twist in me that had to be responsible. If I could only tell the hours, years, the *money* I poured into getting well!"

Finally, a psychiatrist at McLean Hospital in Belmont, Massachusetts, diagnosed Jan as depressed and recommended antidepressants. "Everyone needs a friend," Jan says, "but I think that's where psychotherapy ends—at least for severe depression."

Today there are more than 20 antidepressants on the market, many with fewer side effects than those prescribed a decade ago. Some experts are worried that people will see antidepressants as a quick fix for profoundly complex problems without trying to correct underlying problems through psychotherapy. Others insist that the drugs simply restore a person's emotional equilibrium, allowing problems to be ironed out without the burden of crushing sadness.

"A lot of people didn't do that well in psychotherapy," says psychiatrist Andy Myerson. "It's nice to find solutions in life, but I find that when people take an antidepressant and overcome their depression, they're in a much better position to find the answers to their life's problems themselves."

Iproniazid: The First Antidepressant

The first of the modern antidepressants—iproniazid—was developed in the early 1950s not to treat depression but to ease the symptoms of tuberculosis. At the time, iproniazid was unmatched as a weapon in the ongoing fight against this deadly respiratory illness, decreasing the number of tubercule bacilli and suppressing their proliferation. But while it was designed to treat tuberculosis, as a side benefit iproniazid also seemed to be a sort of "happy drug," pepping up patients, improving their appetites, and restoring their feelings of well-being.

The drug's positive emotional effects immediately attracted the attention of physicians and depression researchers. The only chemical treatment for depression at that time was opium, a highly addictive substance. The possibility of a more effective—and nonaddictive—drug that could alleviate mood disorders was an attractive thought. Up to that time, some drugs could alleviate one or two symptoms of depression, but none could completely eradicate the condition.

Psychiatrists began to consider using iproniazid as a potential antidepressant just when its manufacturers were getting ready to stop production in the wake of newer, even better-acting antitubercular drugs. With the publication of research in 1957 illustrating the success of iproniazid in the treatment of depression, a flurry of prescriptions were written almost immediately. Within that year, physicians had prescribed it for more than 400,000 depressed patients.

Unfortunately, 127 of them developed jaundice. Although historians believe the jaundice was related to viral hepatitis that was epidemic at that time and not to the iproniazid, its manufacturer withdrew the drug because of adverse publicity.

At about the same time, psychiatrist Roland Kuhn began experimenting with imipramine (Tofranil), the first of the cyclic antidepressants. Imipramine was released in 1958, and amitriptyline (Elavil, Endep, and Amitid) was released soon afterward. Eventually, six other tricyclics were introduced in this country.

After reviewing more than 400 clinical studies of antidepressants, a federal panel of researchers concluded that no one antidepressant was clearly more effective than another, and no one drug successfully treated all cases of depression. Only about half of people find relief with the first antidepressant they are prescribed. This panel also found that psychotherapy together with antidepressants is slightly more effective, helping people understand their problems and relieving stress that may worsen symptoms.

How Antidepressants Work

Although scientists don't know for sure, antidepressants appear to correct a chemical imbalance or dysfunction in the brains of depressed people. An antidepressant boosts the level of neurotransmitters important in fighting depression. Each of the major classes of antidepressants— monoamine oxidase inhibitors (MAOIs), tricyclics, and serotonin inhibitors—affects different neurotransmitter systems in a different way.

Tricyclic antidepressants are a class of traditional drugs that treat depression by boosting the level of several different neurotransmitters (norepinephrine, epinephrine, serotonin, and dopamine) by blocking their reabsorption. MAOIs destroy enzymes responsible for burning up neurotransmitters, boosting the neurotransmitter levels. In general, MAOIs are used to treat those who don't respond to tricyclics. Some of the newest antidepressants (including Prozac) interfere with the reabsorption of one specific neurotransmitter (serotonin).

Choosing an Antidepressant

Because it seems as if everyone is talking about Prozac, you may be surprised if your doctor doesn't prescribe it right away for your depression. Actually, many doctors feel more comfortable with one of the older antidepressants (tricyclics or MAOIs) because for more than 35 years they've had success prescribing these drugs.

While these drugs do have more side effects than Prozac and other new drugs, many patients can tolerate these problems. More cautious, conservative physicians may choose an "old reliable" despite miraculous claims for the new medications because of worries about unknown long-term effects. If your doctor gives you one of these older drugs and you can't tolerate the side effects or it doesn't help your depression, then he or she may feel more justified in trying one of the newer drugs.

The complex array of brain chemicals and processes that influence depression tends to differ from one patient to the next; because there's no foolproof way to identify what's causing your depression, prescribing antidepressants may be a trial-and-error process until the right one is found.

"My psychiatrist started me out on Zoloft," recalls Linda, 38. "After six weeks, it had done nothing for me, so he switched me to Wellbutrin. I took that for two weeks, but I became oversensitive. So then I was on Prozac for three days, but it made me manic. Then he tried Paxil and added lithium to keep me from getting manic. That's what I've been on for over a year, and it's been great."

Linda's case illustrates the fact that for many people, the first antidepressant is often not the *right* antidepressant. In fact, only a little more than half of all patients who are given antidepressants find relief with their first prescription. No one is quite sure how or why antidepressants work, and no one can predict who will respond to which drug.

"It's a crapshoot," says Dr. Myerson. "We don't have good guidelines about which person will do well on which drug. So we just have to wade through, try different drugs, adjust dosages, add drugs to drugs. You can have two patients who look identical, but one will respond well to Zoloft and one to Prozac. And we have no idea why."

The best a physician can do is to look at a person's symptoms and try to match those symptoms with an antidepressant. Too often, physicians don't fully explain the side effects and problems a patient may encounter. It's vital to understand the benefits and risks of each antidepressant as you and your physician search for the best treatment.

"Many of my patients don't like to confess that [despite psychotherapy] they are still depressed," one psychiatrist noted. "They feel as if they're letting me down somehow."

There is no one miracle antidepressant that works better than any other, all the time, for everybody. Because depression itself is a complex disease with many causes, doctors must choose from a wide range of antidepressants that work on different brain systems and affect different processes.

When your doctor prescribes an antidepressant be sure you understand:

➤ What drugs might interact with your antidepressant or cause a toxic reaction.

➤ What to do if you miss one dose—or several doses.

➤ The best time of day to take your medication, and how you should take it (on an empty stomach? with food?).

➤ What side effects you should expect and how you should manage them.

➤ How long it will take for the drug to work and how you will know when it's working.

➤ Which side effects are serious enough that you need to contact the doctor immediately.

Combining Drugs

If the first drug fails and your physician has determined that the drug was taken in the right dosage for the correct length of time, he or she may try a different drug. If this second drug also fails, your physician may try combining several different drugs.

When Sara first sought help for her depression, her doctor prescribed an antidepressant and referred her to group therapy. But the first antidepressant didn't seem to do much good—it made her jittery and worsened her sleep problems. When a dosage adjustment didn't improve her symptoms, her psychiatrist switched her to another drug. Sara tried three drugs before finally responding to Zoloft and desipramine, which alleviated her crushing sadness within a few weeks without any other side effects.

Recently, a few psychiatrists—like Sara's doctor—have found that adding desipramine to one of the newer SSRIs such as Prozac or Zoloft seems to work quite well. The dose of each drug is less than would normally be required, so side effects are minimized. A few other drugs, such as thyroid hormone, lithium buspirone (BuSpar), or Ritalin are sometimes added to an MAOI or cyclic antidepressant to boost the drug's effectiveness. While the use of stimulants such as Dexedrine or Ritalin is controversial because of the risk of abuse, adding these drugs to an antidepressant has been successful in alleviating some patients' depression.

If you become psychotically depressed with hallucinations or delusions, your doctor may need to add antipsychotic drugs such as haloperidol (Haldol), thiothixene (Navane), or chlorpromazine (Thorazine) to your antidepressant. Electroconvulsive therapy (ECT) may also be helpful.

Drug combinations can be risky, though, since the more drugs that are given at once, the greater the chance of side effects and drug interactions (such as the dangerous combination of stimulants with MAOIs or certain cyclic antidepressants).

How Long Should You Take Antidepressants?

Length of treatment is becoming controversial. While many people take antidepressants for at least six months to a year, more and more doctors have been suggesting that recurrent depression may be chronic. If you've had more than two episodes of depression, some doctors believe you'll probably need to be on antidepressants for the rest of your life.

On the other hand, it's important not to stop taking antidepressants *too soon*. Research shows that 70 percent of patients become depressed again if they stop taking their antidepressants too early—five weeks or less beyond the point when their symptoms stop. The relapse rate falls to only 14 percent among those who keep taking their antidepressant at least five months after their symptoms abated. Other studies have also found that the longer the patient is on the antidepressant, the less likely is the chance of getting depressed again.

For this reason, many doctors prescribe antidepressants for six months to a year following the end of a depressive episode, gradually tapering off the dosage over several weeks. Unlike opiates, antidepressants aren't addictive, and people taking them will not develop a craving once they are stopped. However, physicians recommend patients gradually taper off the medication to avoid restlessness, anxiety, and other unpleasant physical feelings. This also allows for an opportunity to carefully assess the patient's current need for antidepressant medication.

Side Effects

Side effects from antidepressants generally fall into three categories: sedation; dry mouth, blurry vision, constipation, urinary problems, increased heart rate, and memory problems; and dizziness on standing up (orthostatic hypotension). Drugs that block norepinephrine uptake can produce rapid heartbeat, tremor, and sexual problems. Those that interfere with dopamine (such as Effexor and Asendin) may produce movement disorders and endocrine system changes. Blocking serotonin may create stomach problems, insomnia, and anxiety.

Those that work on the other side of the synapse, blocking receptors that pick up neurotransmitters, have other side effects depending on which receptors are affected. Blocking histamine H_1 receptors produces weight gain and sedation; muscarinic receptor blocks cause dry mouth, constipation, blurry vision, and memory problems.

This is why a tricyclic such as amitriptyline (Elavil) causes so many side effects—it blocks the absorption of both norepinephrine and serotonin, plus four different receptors ($alpha_1$, Dopamine D_2, histamine H_1, and muscarine).

Each drug has a profile of its own particular side effects. Tricyclics often cause dry mouth, constipation, sedation, nervousness, weight gain, and diminished sex drive. MAOIs interact with certain foods and other medications to produce potentially fatal high blood pressure. Newer antidepressants like the SSRIs (such as Prozac, Paxil, and Zoloft) produce fewer side effects than MAOIs or tricyclics because they affect fewer brain pathways, but nausea and headache may occur.

That a drug is characterized by certain side effects doesn't mean you'll necessarily experience any of them; if you do have persistent side effects, you can switch to a drug with a different side-effect profile. Usually, side effects will disappear or diminish in a week or two. In addition, many antidepressants can be taken before bed so the side effects will occur while you sleep. If a bedtime dose makes you too sleepy the next morning, a dose at dinner may be a better idea. A physician can work with your schedule to find the dosage timetable that works best.

Many antidepressants lower sex drive; they might cause impotence or interfere in achieving orgasm. These side effects can be eliminated by adding another drug or changing the antidepressant. In most cases where depression has decreased libido, antidepressants will restore it.

Conclusion

You've just been given a general overview of antidepressants—what they are, how they can help. This book will cover each class of antidepressant, comparing and contrasting them with Prozac and explaining the details of each one.

In the next chapter, you'll learn about the most popular antidepressant ever made—Prozac—and how this little green-and-white pill has changed the face of antidepressant therapy forever.

3

PROZAC

"I realized after taking Prozac that I'd been depressed all my life. I could never really answer the question 'Why do people live? What's the point?' When I was depressed, I couldn't function. A big day was getting the newspaper out of the driveway. Now I'm totally optimistic about everything."

—*Joan, 42, business owner*

It looks ordinary enough, this little green-and-white capsule called Prozac. Not even its manufacturer, Eli Lilly, claims to know exactly why its product works. But more than 10 million people have taken this drug for depression, and more than 70 percent of them have gotten better. Prozac today is the most popular anti-depressant ever.

"I used to walk around with a black cloud over my head," explains Marie, 41. "I was chronically depressed. That's how I felt about life; it was an abyss. But after taking Prozac, my depression is simply gone. I'm not a *different* person, but I'm a *better* person."

If you've had a depressive episode recently, odds are that the first drug your doctor tries will be Prozac (fluoxe-

tine) or one of its cousins, all members of a new antidepressant class called the selective serotonin reuptake
inhibitors (SSRIs). These include Zoloft (sertraline) and
Paxil (paroxetine), Luvox (fluvoxamine), and Serzone
(nefazodone), not an SSRI but a serotonin-related antidepressant.

These drugs have moved to the forefront of modern
psychiatric treatment because they work as well as any of
the older antidepressants while causing far less serious side
effects. Prozac in particular appears to work for a wide
range of other mood disorders in addition to depression.
Your doctor may also recommend Prozac if you suffer
from anxiety or panic disorders, post-traumatic stress, or
eating disorders, although the FDA has approved Prozac
as a treatment only for depression and obsessive-compulsive
disorder. As this book goes to press, the FDA advisory
panel has recommended that Prozac be approved to treat
bulimia, but final approval has not been granted.

How Prozac and Other SSRIs Work

If you lived in a brand-new custom home and a light bulb
burned out on the second-floor landing, you wouldn't
call in an electrician to rip out all the wiring in the walls—
you'd just replace the bulb. There's just no need to disrupt
all the activities in the entire house to fix one simple problem on the second floor.

It's the same way with depression. If you've got a
malfunction in one neurotransmitter system, there's really
no need to take a drug that will interfere with other
neurotransmitter systems and receptor sites throughout

your brain. But for many years, antidepressant drugs did just that.

No one knew how to design a drug that would home in on the light bulb and ignore the wiring in the rest of the house. Yet it appears that some people do seem to get depressed as a result of something as specific as a malfunctioning serotonin system—the neurological equivalent of a burned-out light bulb.

For 10 years, scientists searched for this specific drug, looking at different models of nerve transmission and tailoring chemicals to affect these basic processes. They finally found what they'd been looking for in Prozac. With this chemical, scientists finally had a way to simply replace a burned-out bulb without rewiring the whole house.

The beauty of this new class of drugs is that they're so specific. Unlike the shotgun approach of older drugs like tricyclics (see chapter 5) or monoamine oxidase inhibitors (see chapter 6), which interfere with neurotransmitters and receptor sites all over the brain, Prozac and other SSRIs zero in on serotonin without affecting other brain systems.

The blocking of different neurotransmitters causes different side effects; the greater the number of blocked neurotransmitters, the greater the variety of side effects. For example, blocking the reuptake of norepinephrine can produce tremors, sexual dysfunction, and rapid heart rate. Blocking the reuptake of dopamine can produce movement disorders and changes in the endocrine system. By specifically blocking serotonin alone, you can sidestep most of those problems (although you may still experience stomach upset, insomnia, and anxiety).

In addition, many of the antidepressants also block receptors on the other side of the synaptic gap that normally absorb the neurotransmitters. Blocking one type of receptor causes sedation and weight gain; blocking another type causes blurred vision, dry mouth, constipation, and memory problems.

It now appears that the serotonin neurotransmitter system may be far more complex than anyone had realized, linking areas throughout the brain in an interwoven tapestry of serotonin-producing connections. Not surprisingly, serotonin receptors are especially plentiful in the areas of the brain controlling emotion. What's more, within the past decade, scientists have realized there are at least six different receptor types in the serotonin system, each responsible for sending different signals to different parts of the brain. The next step is to find a drug that can affect just one of these receptor types, and to develop a simple lab test that can identify specific serotonin malfunctions.

While it's apparent that serotonin is of vital importance in the development of depression, scientists aren't so sure that it's a simple cause-and-effect relationship; the brain's biochemical pathways for emotion and mood are just too complex. While it *may* be true that you can directly relieve depression by increasing serotonin, it could be that monkeying around with serotonin causes slight effects in other neurotransmitter systems, and *those* changes relieve depression.

Why Is Prozac So Popular?

Prozac is not really that much different from other SSRIs. So why is Prozac's name on everybody's lips at cocktail parties, widely written about in the media and the topic of countless talk shows?

As the first of the SSRIs to hit the market, by the spring of 1990 Prozac had made the covers of both the *New Yorker* and *Newsweek,* touted as the "new wonder drug for depression." Having heard it praised as a break-through drug that eased depression, had no serious side effects, and helped you lose weight, people began flocking to their family doctors clamoring for prescriptions.

But its early media designation as some sort of happy pill that *every* American might someday want to take to become "better than well" began to raise concerns. Did this drug change behavior, or did it alter personality? It's a sort of chicken-and-egg question that continues to baffle mental health experts. If your mood improves, the outward appearance of your personality and behavior will also change. It stands to reason that if you've been depressed for a long time, you won't have any energy, you might feel negative, you'll mope around, you might have low self-esteem.

If you take Prozac and your depression improves, you begin to feel more positive, and this makes you feel more self-confident. You may begin to take better care of your appearance. It may *seem* that your entire personality changes. But does it? Where does a mood disorder end and personality begin?

If you're a sloppy, negative lout when you're depressed, is that really who you are or just a symptom of your mood disorder? If you can take a pill and alleviate the depression, revealing a buoyant, capable, *healthy* person, is *that* really your true self, or has the pill somehow altered the essential core of your personality?

While Prozac has gotten all the press, experts note that the same process of behavior and personality change occurs with other newly developed antidepressants. It's just that they haven't managed to land on the covers of magazines.

It's also important to note that Prozac won't make healthy people "high" the way marijuana or cocaine might. It won't improve your mood if you're already happy, and if you weren't clinically depressed when you took the pill, odds are Prozac won't do a thing for you.

"I was resistant to seeing Prozac as a cure-all," says Miriam, 26, a Virginia artist. "I never felt it was a lifesaver, but it really did give me a calming effect. It got me out of the house, brought me up from the depths, and removed my feeling of panic."

Miriam said she hated her job as salesclerk and, in a happy relationship for the first time, felt panic as she "waited for it all to fall in. When my emotions reached an overwhelming level, I shuffled from one doctor to another until I saw a psychiatrist, who gave me Prozac."

The idea that prescribing Prozac was a sort of "cosmetic psychopharmacology" was promoted by psychiatrist Peter Kramer, author of the best-selling *Listening to Prozac*. In his book, Kramer expressed concern that this antidepressant alters personality as well as illness in a "substantial minority" of users. Actually, Kramer says he doesn't prescribe Prozac that often and notes that it works for a wide variety of problems in addition to depression. His book was not so much for or against Prozac as it was a philosophical exploration of antidepressants and the human personality.

The fact is that many people in America are looking for a quick fix for minor personality quirks, and others are looking for a safe high. When the media began to imply that anybody could pop a Prozac and eliminate all negative personality traits, these stories naturally created a lot of attention.

Many doctors believe Prozac's reputation as a personality pill has been blown out of proportion. There have been no scientific studies that can back up the claim that Prozac is capable of changing personality *in most people*. It is true, however, that about 10 percent of users will feel much better than they ever did before on this antidepressant—they will feel "better than well."

What Can Prozac Do for You?

About 70 percent of depressed people who take Prozac will experience complete remission within two to six weeks; the rest either don't respond or can't deal with the nausea or insomnia that often occur for the first few days.

Prozac is ideal if you're depressed but sleep normally and need to be able to function during the day. It's also a good choice if you didn't respond to a tricyclic or an MAOI, or if you can't take the side effects of these older drugs. Moreover, if you have weight problems or struggle with obsessions, Prozac might be for you, since studies suggest that people with atypical depression (the symptoms of which include oversleeping and overeating) respond better to Prozac than to tricyclics.

If you don't respond to Prozac, you might do better with one of the older antidepressants (such as the MAOIs or tricyclics), or you might respond to a different SSRI, such as Zoloft or Paxil, or on the just-approved Serzone, a serotonin-related drug. You might also do better on a structurally unrelated antidepressant such as Effexor or Wellbutrin (see chapter 7).

It is also possible that you're one of the very few people who don't respond well to any antidepressant yet on the market.

Should Every Depressed Person Take Prozac?

No. Obviously, if you're allergic to Prozac (look for hives or a rash), you shouldn't take this antidepressant. And if you have serious problems with your liver or kidneys, it's not a good idea to take Prozac because this drug is metabolized in the liver and excreted in the kidneys. If you have serious problems with either of these organs, Prozac could build up in your blood to toxic levels.

You should also be cautious about taking Prozac if you have a history of seizures or epilepsy, even if you're taking anti-seizure medication. Studies of more than 6,000 people revealed that 12 patients experienced seizures with Prozac (a rate of 0.2 percent), about the same rate as that of other antidepressants. If you have such a history, your doctor will want you to have a full neurological workup with an EEG before proceeding. You'll have to take smaller-than-usual doses at first, and you'll probably need a series of EEGs and blood tests (to monitor anticonvulsant levels) during treatment.

Prozac vs. Other SSRIs

What Prozac and all of the other SSRIs do equally well is alleviate depression in most people who try them, without causing a host of unpleasant side effects. This lack of any serious side effects is one reason why physicians are so eager to prescribe the SSRIs, especially for mild depression (dysthymic disorder). Moreover, there has been no evidence of any damage to heart, kidneys, liver, or bone marrow with Prozac.

The main difference between Prozac and other SSRIs is that Prozac stays in the body much longer; this has both positive and negative implications. Prozac's half-life (the time it takes for a drug in the blood to decrease by half of its original dose) is about a week, compared to about a day for Paxil and Zoloft. Up to six weeks after you stop taking the drug, traces of Prozac and its metabolites can still be found in your body. What this means is that if you have a bad reaction to Zoloft or Paxil, the unpleasant symptoms may linger for a week or two. But adverse effects from taking Prozac can last for up to six weeks after you've stopped taking the drug.

There's a benefit to a long half-life, however. You'll be less likely to experience relapse of depression if you forget a dose or two of Prozac, and you'll be less likely to have withdrawal effects from suddenly discontinuing the drug.

Neither Prozac nor the other SSRIs cause the same side effects as older antidepressants—dry mouth, dizziness, blurred vision, constipation. Prozac just helps people feel less fearful, more outgoing, and more self-confident.

Serzone—not an SSRI, but a serotonin-rellated antidepressant—combines the benefits of Prozac with lower price and fewer instances of at least two side effects (insomnia and sexual dysfunction), according to its makers, Bristol-Myers Squibb. While the FDA cautions that no direct comparisons of Serzone have proven its superiority, it does not directly dispute the company's claims. Bristol-Myers Squibb bases its figures on published reports of other drugs' effects.

"Before I took Prozac, every day was difficult," says Joan. "I didn't get any joy out of anything; everything was futile. There seemed to be no hope. After being on Prozac for about a month, I suddenly felt that half my life had already gone by. I'd better get in gear!

"I used to compare myself with everyone," she continues. "Now I don't care. I'm more confident with other people, and I don't freak out in groups. I wish," she sighs, "I had the past 20 years back."

Prozac vs. Older Antidepressants

Not everyone who is depressed experiences the disorder in the same way, and not everyone responds to the same antidepressant.

The main advantage of Prozac, compared with the tricyclics and MAOIs, is that it produces relatively mild side effects.

"Elavil [amitriptyline, a tricyclic] made me tired and stupid, but not less depressed," recalls Marie, who tried a number of antidepressants before responding well to Prozac. "The MAOI was fine, but I couldn't take the diet, and it did weird things to my blood pressure; I kept passing out in inappropriate places. I was in a daze all the time. Of all the drugs I took, Prozac was clearly the best for me. It worked best for the longest period of time, and I didn't have any side effects."

Unlike older antidepressants and lithium, which can be quite toxic, Prozac is not very dangerous even in high doses. Faced with suicidal patients, many doctors feel more comfortable prescribing Prozac, since it's unlikely a person could cause permanent damage by taking too much. (In one case, a patient who supposedly took more than 3,000 milligrams of Prozac did not have lasting physical damage.) Also unlike older antidepressants, it appears to be a good choice if you have heart problems or high blood pressure, since it doesn't appear to affect cardio-vascular function.

Prozac is also a pleasant change for people who just don't like taking pills, since the total daily dose of Prozac can be taken as one capsule or in liquid form, compared with the three to six pills usually needed for MAOIs or tricyclics.

Finally, unlike the many older antidepressants that cause significant weight gain, Prozac doesn't cause weight gain in most people and may even cause them to lose a few pounds. This is partly because of the mild nausea people feel during the first few days, but it's also because Prozac affects the serotonin system and lessens carbohydrate craving. This benefit shouldn't be downplayed, psychiatrists say, since the weight gain caused by the older anti-depressants—which could be 30 pounds or more—could be a real stumbling block to staying on the drug.

This does *not* mean that Prozac is some sort of diet pill. It's more likely to prevent weight gain than to initiate weight loss. Not *everybody* who takes Prozac loses weight, and most only lose a pound or two. One study found that 25 percent of Prozac users did gain weight, although this ratio still compared favorably to the 65 percent of users who gained weight on tricyclics. Researchers note that the heaviest people are those who tend to lose a few pounds on Prozac, while the slimmest users are the ones most likely to gain.

Now for the Down Side

What concerns some doctors—including *Listening to Prozac* author Peter Kramer—is that the drug's long-term effects are largely unknown. A series of studies in humans has shown no connection between antidepressant use and cancer, but there are some concerns about whether antidepressants promote tumor growth in cancer patients or in those exposed to cancer-causing substances (such as nicotine in cigarettes). This concern is primarily due to a small study published in 1992 that found that after being injected with cancer cells or cancer-causing substances, rats subsequently injected with antidepressants had more tumors than control rats.

Cost is also an issue. Older antidepressants like the MAOIs and the tricyclics are cheaper than Prozac and the SSRIs because their patents have expired; they are less expensive compared to these wholesale price tags of some of the newest.

Tolerance is also a concern. (A person develops drug "tolerance" when the drug suddenly stops working, requiring larger and larger doses to be effective.) About one in 50 patients will develop tolerance to any drug, doctors say, and there have been reports of tolerance with Prozac.

Sherry, 38, has suffered for some time with many health problems, including obesity and chronic pain from arthritis. Depressed over these health worries, she began taking one capsule of Prozac daily, which eased her depression at first. She's now up to five tablets daily (100 milligrams), a very high dose indeed.

"The crying episodes have stopped," she reports, "but Prozac is just not very effective anymore. Before, I was always able to pull myself back from depression. Now I'm just crazed, and I've lost faith in traditional medicine."

Some people report strange feelings of loss on Prozac. They feel as if they have changed in some very basic, profound way. They appear to be a little uncomfortable at the thought that while they are not depressed, neither are they *the same person*. Some mental health experts believe this could be the result of suddenly achieving normal mood after years of having adapted as a depressed person.

"What's unsettling is that before, I was internal. I meditated and I prayed a lot," says Jean, 42. "Now that's hard to do. It's hard to hold onto that internal state. I told my doctor I feel shallow. I feel as if I lost an entire dimension of myself. My introspective side has been such a part of me that it's alarming not to be in touch with that side of myself."

Is it disturbing enough to stop taking Prozac? Not to Jean.

"Even if my personality has changed," she says simply, "it's better than being suicidal and living in hell."

This uncomfortable feeling of loss is not unique to Prozac; people taking other SSRIs report similar experiences, especially among those who have battled depression for many years.

"At first, after taking Paxil I didn't know who I was," reports Helen, 39. "It scared me. Relating to people was different, too. When you're depressed, you feel empty inside and you want to fill it up. Once I got un-depressed, I didn't have the neediness that depressed people have. "

Her psychiatrist explained her discomfort very simply. "Helen," he told her, "you've just got to figure out who un-depressed Helen is."

"When I first took Paxil and started feeling better," she says, "I got extremely irresponsible. Before, I worried, worried, worried. Now I just don't care what people think, because I have more self-confidence and self-esteem."

But Helen says she doesn't feel Paxil *changed* her personality at all. "The core of who you are never changes," she explains. "Before I felt sick all over, and now I feel pretty darn good."

Prozac and the other SSRIs can have a profound effect not just on the individual but on his or her family as well. Living with someone who is depressed can be an extremely draining, difficult experience as the mood disorder disrupts everyday family life, dragging others down into depression as well.

Experts in family systems psychology have shown that the successful treatment of anyone in the family will create a sort of ripple effect.

"When I was depressed," says Dan, 43, "I wasn't available to my family. My wife had more of a burden with the kids. I never wanted to go anywhere or do anything. Once I started taking antidepressants, I started enjoying my family again. And *they* started feeling better too. The whole family environment changed for the better."

Drug Interactions

There's nothing wrong with taking both Prozac and over-the-counter pain medications like Tylenol or Advil. And while a few reports suggest that Prozac slows down the rate at which the body breaks down antianxiety drugs such as Valium (diazepam), this doesn't appear to cause any serious problems. Lots of people who are depressed are also anxious, and many people take Valium as part of their treatment. A slowdown in the metabolism rate of Valium simply means the drug will remain in your body for a slightly longer period.

Prozac mixed with tricyclics or a tetracyclic such as Ludiomil isn't dangerous, although Prozac can enhance the effects of these drugs and cause insomnia, appetite loss, and anxiety. And the risk of heart problems and seizure already associated with tricyclics increases when Prozac is added.

But it's *very* dangerous to take Prozac with MAOIs (Nardil, Marplan, or Parnate). This combination could cause a fatal reaction, including nausea and vomiting, high blood pressure and shock. This is why you should wait at least two weeks after taking an MAOI before taking Prozac, and at least five weeks *after* taking Prozac before taking an MAOI.

Combining Other Drugs with Prozac

While you may be started out on a single antidepressant, the current trend in treatment-resistant depression is toward combinations of two medications, either to boost their efficiency or to counteract potential side effects. For example, Desyrel (an antidepressant unrelated to SSRIs or older drugs) is sometimes added to Prozac if a patient has trouble sleeping when taking Prozac alone.

"I take Desyrel right before I go to sleep," says Sarah, 42. "Before taking antidepressants, I was having a lot of trouble sleeping because of my depression. But Prozac didn't help that. So after a few weeks on Prozac, my psychiatrist added Desyrel, and I started sleeping again for the first time in years."

Some research suggests that a combination of Prozac and lithium may help some people who don't improve on either drug alone.

What About Those Suicide Reports?

There's an ongoing controversy about whether Prozac causes people to try to kill themselves, or whether suicide attempts by users of Prozac are the result of the depression itself.

Studies have shown that at the beginning of treatment, 10 percent to 15 percent of patients feel more anxious after taking Prozac, but this anxiety eventually passes.

There also have been reports of anger and irritability among users of Prozac. Very irritable patients usually find their temperaments improving on Prozac, but it's a different story with manic-depressives. If manic highs involve anger, paranoia, or irritability and you take Prozac without first being stabilized on lithium, the manic side of your mood may break through and you could experience these symptoms. Many scientists believe that Prozac may initially increase manic symptoms because the drug increases a person's energy *before* it has successfully altered mood. This could suddenly prompt a suicide attempt in someone who had previously been too lethargic to make the effort. Indeed, several studies have suggested that people who are slowed down by depression in this way do appear to have a temporary increased risk of suicide as the depression eases.

Prozac experienced a temporary backlash in 1990 after reports circulated that it induced violent and suicidal tendencies in some users; the Church of Scientology led the attack against the drug, which focused on a small group of patients who had suicidal or violent thoughts. In 1990 the church filed a citizen's petition with the U.S. Food and Drug Administration asking that Prozac be withdrawn from the market, citing a Harvard Medical School study published in the *American Journal of Psychiatry* stating that 6 out of 172 high-risk mental patients who had been resistant to other drugs had become preoccupied with violent suicidal thoughts while on Prozac. Two of them tried unsuccessfully to kill themselves. Although none of the six had appeared to be suicidal when they started taking Prozac, five had had suicidal thoughts before. At the time, four of the six were also taking other medications (one was taking five other drugs).

The Scientologists took that study's findings of the six individuals and extrapolated them to the entire United States population, claiming that 140,000 people in the

United States have become violent and suicidal on Prozac and charging that widespread use of Prozac would promote waves of violence. They backed up this claim by pointing to mass murderer Joseph Wesbecker, who killed himself and eight coworkers at a printing plant in Louisville, Kentucky, with an AK-47 assault rifle. A Scientology group alleged that Wesbecker, who they said had no history of violence, went berserk because he took Prozac. Subsequent media reports revealed Wesbecker had a large gun collection, had tried to kill himself 12 times in the past, and had often talked about killing his employers.

Because so many depressed people are also suicidal, the fact that a few severely depressed patients taking antidepressants became suicidal didn't surprise researchers. The FDA *was* concerned, however, because Prozac affects serotonin, a neurotransmitter known to be linked with aggression. After further study, however, in 1991 the FDA rejected the petition, reaffirming Prozac's safety. This decision was followed two months later by a unanimous announcement by the FDA advisory committee and an independent scientific advisory committee that Prozac and other antidepressants do not cause violence or suicidal behavior, and that Prozac, on the contrary, appears to guard *against* violent behavior. The announcement included the information that large-scale studies show that people taking Prozac are less suicidal than those taking a placebo or other antidepressant drugs. This affirmation of support was backed by the National Mental Health Association and the American Psychiatric Association.

The research the groups relied on included an extremely large comparison of 3,065 patients on antidepressants published in the *British Medical Journal*. The study found no evidence of increased suicide risk or suicidal thoughts in people taking Prozac or tricyclics. In the study, Prozac caused fewer substantial suicidal thoughts than did tricyclics or placebo. Of those people who did have suicidal thoughts when they started taking the drugs, those given a placebo had the highest increase in those thoughts, with Prozac showing the least increase (17.9 percent for placebo, 16.3 percent for tricyclics and 15.3 percent for Prozac). Most patients taking Prozac and tricyclics experienced a *decrease* in suicidal thoughts (about 72 percent).

By January 1994, 78 suits against Eli Lilly (Prozac's manufacturers) had been dismissed and 160 others had been filed, charging that Prozac causes everything from rashes to violent death.

"When I first went on Prozac, it was in the early days when everyone was talking about suicide and this drug," Marie says. "I was somewhat concerned about that. My friends asked me if I was sure I knew what I was doing."

Indeed, despite the suits and bad publicity, the popularity of this drug never declined; Lilly's Prozac sales haven't had a bad year since the drug was released in 1987. In 1993, sales reached $1.2 billion worldwide ($880 million in the United States alone), surpassing the sales of all previously used antidepressants around the world. Sales are expected to increase another 12 percent in 1994.

As we've seen from the above discussion, if you're depressed, it's possible you might have some suicidal thoughts; between 40 and 60 percent of people with major depression do. *Tell your doctor immediately if you start feeling self-destructive.*

How Prozac Is Administered

You'll probably be started out on 10 to 20 milligrams daily, and if you haven't responded within a month, your dosage may be increased to as much as 40 milligrams. Most patients don't take more than 80 milligrams, however, and some studies suggest that lower doses usually work better. (In a few cases, very obese people have responded to doses over 80 milligrams although this excessive dosage is not recommended in general because of safety concerns.)

Like all antidepressants, Prozac doesn't work overnight. It will usually take two to three weeks before you start to notice a difference in how you're feeling, although some people insist their depression improves within the first week. In most cases, depression lifts within one to two months. You should take the full dose for at least six weeks before deciding that it's not going to work. If you do have a good response, most doctors recommend you continue taking Prozac for six to eight months before stopping. If you're contemplating stopping, it's better to wait until you appear to have no upcoming stress, such as divorce proceedings or a major sales presentation. When you and your doctor decide it's time to stop taking Prozac, your doctor will teach you how to tell if your depression is returning.

Withdrawal

Unlike a few other antidepressants, Prozac produces no withdrawal symptoms when you stop taking it. Because of its long half-life, you can stop taking Prozac abruptly without complications. However, some doctors suggest you taper off your doses and closely watch for any indication of a relapse.

If you begin to feel lethargic, have low moods, or experience appetite or sleep problems, your depression could be returning. *These are not the symptoms of any sort of withdrawal.* If it is your depression returning, you can start taking Prozac again and it should work as well as it did before.

Unfortunately, some people do experience depression again and again. Because of the underlying biological component of depression, there's at least a 50-percent chance you may experience another episode. For those who've already had two episodes, the chances of a third jump to about 90 percent. Therefore, for cases of recurrent depression, experts today sometimes recommend taking Prozac indefinitely to prevent future occurrences.

Side Effects

The most frequent complaint about Prozac is nausea; you may not feel very hungry for the first few days. But this nausea usually disappears after about two weeks. It may help to take your medication with a meal, or to divide your dose in half for awhile; ask your doctor about this.

But if your nausea doesn't go away in a week or two, or it gets worse, you may have to switch to another antidepressant.

Other common side effects include nervousness and anxiety. Prozac can be very stimulating, and some people feel a caffeine-like buzz after first taking this drug. "When I take Prozac, I feel jittery," Joan says, "sort of like drinking five pots of coffee. Other than that, I don't have any physical side effects."

Prozac's stimulatory properties also can cause sleep problems in some people, probably because Prozac (like other SSRIs) affects serotonin, responsible for regulating the sleep-wake cycle. Fortunately, only about 2 percent of patients find the insomnia so troubling that they are forced to stop taking Prozac. About the same percentage are equally disturbed by drowsiness with this drug. If you do experience insomnia, you can try taking your medicine earlier in the day, or ask your doctor about combining Prozac with Desyrel (trazodone).

About 9 percent of people taking Prozac report dry mouth, compared to about 65 percent of those taking tricyclics. A few people also notice sweating, tremors, or rash.

Most antidepressants (except for Wellbutrin) cause some degree of sexual problems, and Prozac isn't any different. As many as 40 percent of people experience some negative sexual effects, including delayed ejaculation, impotence, decreased desire, or problems reaching orgasm. Patients cite loss of sexual interest as one of the biggest problems with Prozac. On the other hand, some people feel *more* interested in sex than before, possibly because depression had interfered with their libido.

More seriously, Prozac can induce a manic state (excess elation, hyperactivity, agitation, and speeded-up

thinking and talking) in people who are inclined to be
manic-depressive. This is a real problem, and it's something your doctor will be watching out for, especially if
there's a history of manic depression in your family. Your
doctor may want to cut back your dose or combine

SIDE EFFECTS OF PROZAC

Most common (in order of frequency)
    Sexual dysfunction (40 percent)
    Nausea (21 percent)
    Headache (20 percent)
    Insomnia (14 percent)
    Diarrhea or drowsiness (12 percent)

Less common (10 percent or fewer patients)
    Anxiety
    Dry mouth
    Appetite loss
    Tremor
    Upper respiratory infection
    Dizziness

Infrequent (fewer than 5 percent)
    Fatigue
    Constipation
    Abdominal pain
    Flulike symptoms
    Vision problems
    Congestion
    Sinus infection
    Cough
    Mania

Prozac with lithium to manage the mania. Some people may have to stop the drug completely.

"Prozac made me speed," says Julie, a 38-year-old woman with a family history of manic depression. "I was scouring every nook and cranny. I had two vacuums going in the bedroom at once, one for the corners and one for the floor. I hadn't cleaned that much for two years, because I was depressed. Once I took Prozac, suddenly I felt like doing a *really good job*. The night before I went on the cleaning binge, I lay in bed for two hours thinking that I could smell the dust. As soon as I told my psychiatrist, he immediately took me off Prozac and put me on Paxil."

What If You're Pregnant or Breast-feeding?

Animal studies haven't found any problems with taking Prozac during pregnancy, even in 10 times the normal human dosage. However, animals and people sometimes react differently.

A study in the January 1997 *New England Journal of Medicine* concluded that taking Prozac or tricyclic antidepressants during pregnancy doesn't affect the IQ, language development, or behavior of the child, at least throughout the preschool years. In a study of more than 200 preschoolers, there also were no significant differences in temperament, mood, activity level, distractibility, or other problems, according to researchers at the University of Toronto in Ontario, Canada. Moreover, there were no developmental differences between infants who were exposed to antidepressants only during the first three months of pregnancy and those whose mothers took the drugs throughout pregnancy.

Previous research has shown that infants who were exposed to the antidepressants in the womb were no more likely to have major birth defects than those who were never exposed. Although one study indicated taking Prozac during the third trimester of pregnancy might lower an infant's birth weight and increase the risk of preterm delivery, the new study found no evidence of such problems.

At the time the children were born and when they were tested for learning and behavioral problems, their weights, and heights were similar regardless of whether their mothers had taken an antidepressant during pregnancy. Moreover, the study found that women who had taken the drugs during pregnancy were no more likely to give birth prematurely than those who hadn't taken them.

Because depression during pregnancy is a big problem, birthing experts felt reassured that at last there are some reassuring data about the safety of these drugs. Untreated depression can have a negative effect on pregnancy, especially if a woman has problems eating or sleeping.

While this study is encouraging, experts really can't be certain yet about the safety and effects of antidepressant use during pregnancy Most doctors recommend that, if at all possible, you not use Prozac (or any other antidepressant) if you're pregnant or trying to conceive. However, if you become severely depressed without medication during pregnancy, you and your must weigh the severity of the depression with the available information on how the drug might affect a developing fetus.

Like most antidepressants, Prozac is secreted in mother's milk. Since scientists just don't know what effect this might have on the baby, most doctors recommend that you not plan to breast-feed if you're taking Prozac. You'll need to weigh these decisions, however, since Prozac and many other antidepressants *are* effective in treating postpartum depression.

Prozac and Youth

While antidepressants have not been widely studied in children, a few studies suggest children and adolescents may be given Prozac provided they are carefully screened for manic depression in themselves or their family.

Because Prozac doesn't appear to cause the cardio-vascular problems in children that sometimes occur with other antidepressants, some doctors find this a good choice. And Prozac has proven to be very effective against both bulimia—so troubling in adolescence—and obsessive-compulsive disorder, which often appears in childhood.

Studies suggest younger people respond with very small doses, possibly as small as 5 to 10 milligrams daily to start. Studies also show that a sizable portion of young people who do not respond to other antidepressants do respond to Prozac.

Studies also suggest that younger people experience slightly different side effects than those experienced by older patients. Restlessness and sweating are the most commonly reported side effects, together with drowsiness, dry mouth, tremors, and thinning hair.

Prozac and the Elderly

If you're over 65 and depressed, chances are you'll respond just as well to Prozac as you would to a number of other antidepressants (such as nortriptyline, a tricyclic antidepressant). However, because side effects like dry mouth and constipation aren't such a problem with Prozac and the other SSRIs, you're more likely to be able to tolerate treatment. And, as we've discussed above, Prozac is ideal for older people because it doesn't interfere with blood pressure or heart function. In fact, Prozac and the other SSRIs (plus Wellbutrin) are among the safest antidepressants for people with heart disease. For these reasons, more and more psychiatrists are reaching for Prozac and other SSRIs for their older patients.

There have been a few reports noting that some older people taking Prozac have low levels of sodium in their blood, causing them to retain water, which can lead to swelling. Your doctor will advise you if you are likely to experience this problem.

Prozac and Obsessive-Compulsive Disorder

Since Prozac affects the serotonin system, and because serotonin has been implicated in a host of other disorders, it's not surprising that Prozac appears to help lots of other problems besides depression.

In July 1993, the FDA approved Prozac for the treatment of obsessive-compulsive disorder. This disorder is surprisingly common in this country, affecting 5 million Americans with symptoms commonly beginning as early as age 10.

People with OCD become obsessed with certain thoughts and bogged down with repetitive activities like washing their hands or rechecking doors and windows. (A "compulsion" is a rigid behavior that is repeated over and over every day.) If you have OCD, you may be fearful about dirt, disease, or toxic chemicals, or you may need to count, align, check, or apologize constantly.

People with OCD are not out of touch with reality. They *know* their behavior isn't reasonable, and about a third are so upset about their problem that they become clinically depressed.

Studies have shown that Prozac can help up to 70 percent of these people, although it can take up to 10 weeks to notice improvement. Patients usually take higher doses of Prozac for OCD on a long-term basis. And because Prozac does not carry many of the harmful side effects that interfere with antidepressant use in children, it has been given to young OCD patients with favorable results. One study reported that four out of eight young-sters given up to 80 milligrams of Prozac daily completely stopped their handwashing rituals after two months.

The SSRI Luvox (fluvoxamine) and the tricyclic Anafranil (clomipramine) are also very effective treatments.

Prozac and Eating Disorders

Bulimia

Prozac has been approved by the FDA advisory committee for the treatment of bulimia, a sometimes-fatal disorder of compulsive eating binges and self-induced vomiting and laxative abuse. Estimates of bulimia sufferers range from

1 percent to 10 percent of all American women and up to 14 percent of college-age women.

Some research suggests that depression can be an underlying cause of eating disorders; one study of bulimics found that three out of four bulimic patients were depressed.

Studies suggest that Prozac can help ease eating binges in up to 63 percent of people with bulimia nervosa. While MAOIs also help with bulimia, the side effects and rigid diet restrictions often cause problems for patients. And because many patients taking MAOIs gain weight, the chance is small that patients will stick with this medication regimen considering their intolerable fear of weight gain. In fact, a recent study of 27 bulimic patients found that while they responded well to the drug, 24 stopped taking the drug within four months because of the side effects.

Some scientists believe that Prozac may be helpful in correcting bulimia because it reduces appetite; some studies found that rats given fluoxetine and then deprived of their favorite food for a day ate less than they would normally eat. Other experts believe the drug corrects the underlying serotonin malfunction, pointing out that other antidepressants that don't affect appetite but do affect serotonin are also effective against bulimia.

In another study, up to 65 percent of bulimic patients responded to antidepressants, although many did not respond to the first drug that was tried. In this particular study, 6 of the 17 patients who experienced remission of their symptoms were taking Prozac.

A combination of psychotherapy and Prozac has been the most effective treatment for bulimia.

Anorexia nervosa

Anorexic patients have antidepressant needs that are a little different from bulimic subjects. Still, a new study by the University of Pittsburgh Medical Center found that Prozac

---

OTHER DISORDERS AND PROZAC

Prozac has also been used to treat a wide variety of other disorders; studies have shown that at least some people have improved when taking Prozac for PMS, nicotine withdrawal, exhibitionism, dementia, Tourette's syndrome, and even itchy skin under certain circumstances. Some of the more common disorders that are being treated with Prozac include:

PREMENSTRUAL SYNDROME
Surveys have shown that between 3 and 8 percent of North American women suffer from premenstrual syndrome. Recent studies have shown what physicians have already found to be true—many women find relief from symptoms when taking Prozac.

A recent Canadian study of 180 women found that half of the subjects taking Prozac daily for six months had at least a moderate improvement in their symptoms. By contrast, only 22 percent of those taking a placebo reported a moderate decrease in symptoms. In addition, significantly more women taking the Prozac reported better than 75 percent improvement in their symptoms, and both small (20 mg) and large doses (60 mg) were equally effective. The smaller dose, however, caused fewer side effects (nausea, fatigue, dizziness, and concentration problems).

While it is not clear why PMS responds to Prozac, scientist note that many of the features of PMS are similar to those of depression.

BODY DYSMORPHIC DISORDER
People with body dysmorphic disorder (the false perception that a part of the body is abnormal) generally feel better with a SSRI.

ALCOHOLISM
Several studies have found that Prozac may help alcoholics decrease the amount of alcohol they drink, while other SSRIs increased the number of days alcoholics can abstain from drinking.

PANIC ATTACKS

If you've ever experienced the frightening wave of panic common to
those with panic disorder, you'll be happy to hear that many patients
respond to Prozac. In one study, about half of people with panic
attacks become free of panic after taking Prozac, while the other half
reported they become *more* anxious with this drug. Another study
found that seven of eight people with panic disorders found complete
relief with Prozac. A third found that 19 out of 25 panic patients
showed moderate to remarkable improvement. And by reducing panic,
it's possible also to ease the *agoraphobia* (fear of being in places where
they feel vulnerable) that often is associated with panic attacks.
Behavioral therapy together with Prozac or another antidepressant may
be the best treatment for panic attacks.

MENTAL DISORDERS

Studies suggest that Prozac can improve functioning in patients suffering from either schizophrenia or borderline personality disorder.
Schizophrenics, for example, may become less aggressive and more
interested in social activities.

can help patients with anorexia. When 16 women with
the eating disorder were given Prozac, 10 stayed at a
healthy weight and didn't relapse, while only three of 19
anorexic women placed on a placebo were able to remain
healthy. This study is the first to show an antidepressant
could help prevent anorexia relapses, according to study
director Walter Kaye, M.D. Prozac may help by altering
brain chemicals that affect both mood and appetite.
Experts were hopeful because a medication that can help
patients maintain a healthy weight outside of a hospital and
prevent relapse can ultimately save lives. Currently, there is
no anorexia treatment that has been approved by the FDA.

What Prozac and other antidepressants can do is to
address the underlying biological problem that may be
causing the eating disorder; this treatment, combined

with supportive psychotherapy and nutritional counseling, may help break the cycle of anorexia.

Conclusion

In this chapter, we've seen that Prozac is not some sort of wonder drug, happy pill, or panacea. It's about as effective as any other antidepressant, without many of the harmful side effects.

Perhaps the best result of the incredible wave of media interest and public fascination with this medication is that it has set off a widespread discussion of depression itself, together with the idea that *it can be treated successfully.*

But keep in mind that there are several other new antidepressants in the same class (SSRIs) that are just as effective as Prozac. For reasons we don't yet understand, some people respond better to one than another. We'll discuss these new alternatives, including Zoloft, Paxil, and Serzone, in the next chapter.

4

SELECTIVE SEROTONIN REUPTAKE INHIBITORS

"When I was depressed, I lost interest in life. For three months I didn't open my mail. My driver's license was revoked and I didn't even know it. People don't understand that there are real consequences to being so depressed that you can't take care of everyday business."
—Verna, 42

Angela, 70, was under a lot of stress at home that just kept getting worse. She and her husband had moved to a smaller apartment, and her husband had been diagnosed with prostate cancer. For the past three months, she'd been feeling more and more depressed and anxious. She'd begun to lose weight; she couldn't concentrate; she felt helpless and worthless. To her husband's alarm, she began talking about suicide. Deeply concerned, they finally sought help for her at a psychiatric hospital.

Four days after getting a prescription for Zoloft (sertraline) and beginning psychotherapy, she was back home. In three weeks, she was back to her normal self and was no longer troubled by the same problems that had seemed so difficult only a few weeks before. Angela's suicidal thoughts had disappeared.

After six months, Zoloft and her therapy were stopped, and one year later the depression had not returned.

In the previous chapter on Prozac, we presented an overview of how the SSRIs work. In this chapter, we will discuss the *other* SSRIs, Zoloft and Paxil, and the newest serotonin-related drug, Serzone. The other serotonin-related drug, Luvox, should be approved soon by the FDA for the treatment of depression.

Prime Candidates

The SSRIs are particularly helpful in heading off depression in the early stages, before it becomes deeply rooted. Recent studies suggest that SSRIs are ideal for those people with minor depressive illness—much better than tricyclics, such as imipramine, or the complication-prone MAOIs. The SSRIs are certainly effective for major depression, too.

"Before taking Zoloft, I had a bad case of the blahs. Everything just seemed colorless. But now, sometimes I'll just lie in bed and rub the blanket between my fingers," says Sharon, 38. "It's not sexual, but my sensitivity is heightened. The feel-goodness goes right down into my bones."

Research seems to suggest that you can head off serious full-blown illness by taking an SSRI during the early stages of depression. These drugs work so well that someday soon, doctors may begin recommending early screening for depression, just as they now recommend early screening for breast cancer and high blood pressure.

This doesn't mean that SSRIs are the *only* worth-while antidepressant, of course. There is still a place for the older drugs.

Researchers note that the SSRIs don't work for 20 percent to 40 percent of depressed or anxious people who try them—the same failure rate as for the older antidepressants.

Which SSRI Is Best?

Most experts agree that no single SSRI is better than the rest, despite Prozac's recent image as a miracle drug that not only cures depression but can make many healthy people "better than well" (see chapter 3). Each drug has a certain profile of its own particular side effects; some have markedly similar side effects, while others vary widely.

For example, Zoloft and Paxil don't last as long in the body as Prozac; the half-life of Zoloft is about 26 hours, and the half-life of Paxil is about 21 hours. ("Half-life" is the time it takes for a drug in the blood to decrease by half of its original dose.)

It's important to understand that all the SSRIs may cause nausea, headache, anxiety, dry mouth, insomnia, and a variety of sexual dysfunctions. But as mentioned, what makes Prozac less desirable is that it lingers in the body much longer than other SSRIs; up to six weeks after you stop taking the drug, traces of Prozac and its metabolites can still be found in your body. If you have a bad reaction to Zoloft or Paxil, symptoms last for a week or two. But side effects while taking Prozac can last for up to six weeks before all traces of the drug leave your body.

Of course, none of the SSRIs are any sort of wonder drug. They all have some side effects, although they are less severe than those of other antidepressants.

One of the biggest problems with these drugs is their cost. All of them are much more expensive than the generic versions of older drugs like MAOIs or tricyclics. Generic versions of the older drugs are available because their patents have expired.

No matter how wonderful a drug may be, if you can't afford it, it's not going to do you much good. The high cost of the SSRIs can be a real hardship for someone with no insurance, or whose insurance doesn't cover drugs. At about $2 to $3 per pill, the pharmacy bill can be overwhelming.

It's a problem for Mary, 28, whose health insurance covers all drugs *except* medications for mental health problems. "My psychiatrist is very aware of this problem," Mary explains. "He doesn't give me Zoloft alone because it would be too expensive. So he prescribes a smaller amount of Zoloft with desipramine (a less-expensive tricyclic)." The desipramine boosts the effects of Zoloft, and the combination costs less than a full dose of Zoloft alone.

Serotonin-Related Drugs

Serzone is the first of a new type of antidepressant manufactured by Bristol-Myers Squibb that has been approved by the FDA and is chemically different from other antidepressants.

Serzone combines the main mechanisms of two major classes of drugs—the SSRIs and the tricyclics—with fewer instances of at least two problematic side effects (insomnia and sexual dysfunction).

However, the FDA has cauutioned that direct comparisons between Serzone and other antidepressants have not yet been done, although it does not directly dispute the company's claims. Bristol-Myers bases its claims on figres in puublished reports of other drugs' side effects.

Serzone is the first drug that boosts the brains' level of serotonin while blocking serotonin receptors. While clinical trials have found Serzone to be as effective at alleviating depression as other drugs, when taken twice a day it shows little problems of disturbing sleep. As many as one in five patients taking an SSRI are also prescribed some type of sleep aid.

Sexual dysfunction may occur in SSRI users from one to five percent according to the drug companies (although actual incidence of the problem may be much higher, critics charge—as high as 40 percent). The incidence of sexual problems among Serzone patients is cited at 1.5 percent, according to Bristol-Myers.

Medical Cautions

Severe kidney or liver disease could result in higher-than-normal blood levels of the SSRIs. In addition, the SSRIs may not be the best choice in the treatment of patients with mania, or in those with a history of seizures.

Side Effects

The side effects of SSRIs are usually mild and manageable, although once in a while a sensitive person gets a severe reaction. Like most antidepressants, SSRIs may cause nausea, dizziness, or dry mouth, not to mention a range of sexual-function side effects, including decreased sexual interest (in men), increased sexual interest (in women), ejaculation problems, impotence, or menstrual changes.

The most common side effects with Zoloft, launched in 1991, and Paxil, introduced in 1993, are insomnia, diarrhea, tremor, and drowsiness. If you get side effects while taking either of these, your doctor may switch you to Wellbutrin, as long as you don't have any of the conditions that might make you vulnerable to seizures with this drug (such as previous severe head injury or epilepsy). And like Prozac, Zoloft and Paxil can produce mild mania in some people with a genetic tendency in that direction.

Luvox (fluvoxamine) is an SSRI recently approved by the FDA for the treatment of obsessive-compulsive disorder but not yet approved for depression in this country. (It has been used as an antidepressant for several years in Europe and Canada.)

Drug Interactions

Given together, tryptophan and any of the SSRIs may cause headache, nausea, sweating, and dizziness. Taking an SSRI within two weeks of an MAOI (such as Marplan or Parnate) may cause serious side effects; you should wait at least two weeks between stopping MAOIs and starting an SSRI, or at least five weeks after stopping an SSRI and starting an MAOI.

Combining Paxil and warfarin may cause excess bleeding. If you're taking cimetidine, which can cause an increase in the blood levels of Paxil, your dosage of Paxil should be adjusted.

Research suggests that Zoloft, unlike MAOIs or tricyclics, doesn't necessarily appear to cause problems when mixed with alcohol. However, Zoloft's manufacturers don't recommend the combination.

There are no known dangerous reactions between nonprescription drugs and Zoloft, but because it's theoretically possible, be sure to talk to your doctor about any other drugs you take. Combining Zoloft with either digitoxin (Crystodigin) or warfarin (Coumadin) may cause unwanted side effects.

Pregnancy and Breast-feeding

Most SSRIs haven't been studied in nursing mothers or pregnant women, but animal studies have suggested that Zoloft may cause developmental problems or decrease survival of offspring. Animal studies with Paxil haven't revealed any birth defects.

Other Disorders

The SSRIs may be an effective treatment for other disorders besides depression. Luvox appears to be as effective as Prozac or clomipramine for obsessive-compulsive disorder. Paxil has been approved by the FDA for obsessive-compulsive disorder and panic disorder. Zoloft has been approved for obsessive-compulsive disorder.

Withdrawal

Research with SSRIs has *not* found that people become dependent on the drug or have withdrawal symptoms when they stop taking it. Nevertheless, you should let your doctor know if you develop any troubling symptoms while taking, or after stopping, an SSRI.

Conclusion

We've seen how the SSRIs have transformed the treatment of depression by offering a choice of several drugs with low toxicity and few side effects. Unfortunately, not everyone responds to these new drugs; for some people, older antidepressants such as the tricyclics are far more effective. In chapter 5, we'll explore the development of the tricyclics, the very first antidepressants, plus a later development known as the tetracyclic.

5

CYCLIC ANTIDEPRESSANTS

"What I remember most about being depressed was always being exhausted. I could never get to sleep at night, and when I did, I had nightmares. Then I'd wake up in the morning and have to drag myself to work. And in all that time—four or five years, I guess—I never once enjoyed anything. I was actually planning my own suicide when my doctor referred me to a psychiatrist who put me on imipramine. For the first time in years, I finally began to get some pleasure out of life."

—Sam, 43

Before Prozac, tricyclics were the first line of defense against encroaching depression, and had been ever since imipramine's release in 1958 under the brand name Tofranil. Today, tricyclics are a less popular choice than the new generation of antidepressants, but they're still an important weapon in the antidepressant arsenal for a subset of people who don't respond to anything else.

Before tricyclics were developed, psychiatrists treating severely depressed clients had only two real choices: amphetamines or electroshock therapy. Imipramine was

COMMON CYCLIC ANTIDEPRESSANTS
(Lower doses are used with elderly patients)

DRUG	USUAL EFFECTIVE DAILY DOSE
Amitriptyline (Elavil, Endep, Emitrip, Enovil)	150–300 mg
Amoxapine (Asendin)	150–400 mg
Clomipramine (Anafranil)	100–150 mg
Desipramine (Norpramin, Pertofrane)	100–300 mg
Doxepin (Adapin, Sinequan)	75–300 mg
Imipramine (Janimine, Tipramine, Tofranil, Tofranil-PM)	150–300 mg
Maprotiline (Ludiomil)	75–150 mg
Nortriptyline (Pamelor, Aventyl)	50–150 mg
Protriptyline (Vivactil)	15–60 mg

discovered by Swiss scientists searching for a successful schizophrenia treatment; it turned out that imipramine didn't do much for schizophrenia at all. What it *did* do very well was perk up depressed patients.

With the discovery of imipramine, doctors finally had a drug that relieved a person's underlying depression. And when scientists realized how effective imipramine was—about 70 percent of depressed patients responded to this drug—they flocked to the laboratories in search of similar drugs based on imipramine's three-ring ("tricyclic") antihistaminic chemical structure. Before long, laboratories all over the country began churning out tricyclic clones, each one a little different from, but none any better than, imipramine itself. A later-developed drug in this class, maprotiline (Ludiomil), had four rings and was therefore called "tetracyclic." Taken together, the tricyclics and tetracyclics are known as "heterocyclics" or "cyclics."

But while all these cyclics were effective, not one provided the perfect solution to depression for which scientists had been searching.

How They Work

The cyclic antidepressants work by beefing up the brain's supply of norepinephrine and serotonin levels—chemicals that are abnormally low in depressed patients. This allows the flow of nerve impulses to return to normal. The cyclics do *not* act by stimulating the central nervous system or by blocking monoamine oxidase.

The problem with cyclics is that they don't stop there. They go on to interfere with a range of other neurotransmitter systems and a variety of brain cell receptors, affecting nerve cell communication all over the brain in the process. And the more neurotransmitter systems and receptors you affect, the more side effects a patient will have.

Who Responds to Cyclics

Side effects notwithstanding, for some people the cyclics work better than any other drug available.

"I've been taking imipramine for the past five years," says Carol, 47, a New Jersey teacher. "It was the first and only antidepressant I've ever taken. When I was depressed, I had a feeling of being lost. I was discontented with myself—I felt 'blah' for a long time. I just don't feel that way anymore."

The challenge, of course, is to figure out *who* will respond best to them. The important thing to understand is that some types of tri- and tetracyclics are riskier than others, and some people tolerate some types better.

Just as scientists aren't sure exactly what causes depression, they're not sure exactly what cures it, either. Often, your doctor will choose an antidepressant drug for you based not on the cause of your depression as much as the symptoms you have, and how well you might be expected to tolerate certain side effects.

Unfortunately, there's no simple test that can reveal which drug might work best for you. How well you react to any particular drug is often as much a surprise to your doctor as it is to you. That's why it may take some time before you and your doctor discover the perfect antidepressant "fit."

The tricyclic nortriptyline (Pamelor), for example, may be useful in treating patients with depression following a stroke.

Both trimipramine and imipramine work equally well at relieving depression in hospitalized patients. Because it has a sedative effect, the tetracyclic Ludiomil is useful in treating depression accompanied by anxiety or sleeping problems. Protriptyline is more likely to aggravate agitation and anxiety, but it's particularly good if you're withdrawn or lethargic and tired. On the other hand, it's likely to cause sleeping problems, especially when taken late in the day. (For this reason, protriptyline is a popular choice in the treatment of narcolepsy.)

In the past, depressed patients were almost always started out on tricyclics. With the growing popularity of SSRIs, however, most patients are now given Prozac or Zoloft, and then moved to a tricyclic or tetracyclic if the depression doesn't respond to the first- or second-choice drugs.

"When I became very depressed after experiencing some family problems, I tried Prozac," reports Gina, 52, a personnel manager in Arizona. "But after six months it hadn't affected my depression at all. So my doctor switched me to imipramine. Within a few weeks, I felt less prone to tears, less hopeless. It's not so much that I was suddenly pro-life. It's just that the negative outlook wasn't so stupefying."

Sometimes, doctors may add Prozac or lithium to small doses of tri- or tetracyclics to boost the antidepressants' effectiveness. However, this can be risky; the combination has sometimes caused an increase in the blood level of the cyclic. Since cyclics already can be dangerous to the heart and can set off seizures, adding Prozac may increase this risk.

Who Shouldn't Take Cyclics

The first job for your doctor is to decide whether you're one of the people who *shouldn't* take cyclic antidepressants. Obviously, your doctor won't prescribe them if you're allergic to this type of antidepressant. If you've taken an MAOI within the past two weeks, you'll want to wait two weeks before taking cyclics, since the combination of these two can cause serious side effects.

If you have any kind of drinking problem, you should avoid cyclics, since alcohol can be toxic when mixed with these drugs.

Schizophrenics or manic-depressives shouldn't take cyclics, since these drugs can worsen the symptoms of schizophrenia and may push a depressed manic-depressive into a manic state if the person isn't already taking an anti-manic medication (such as lithium).

There are also some specific health problems that don't mix well with certain antidepressants. If you have a problem with your bone marrow function or any blood cell disorder or if you have seizures or an adrenalin-producing tumor, you'll want to stay away from clomipramine (Anafranil).

If you have serious heart disease, you should avoid trimipramine (Surmontil). Ludiomil shouldn't be used if you have a seizure disorder, or if you've had a heart attack within the past six weeks.

You should also avoid Ludiomil if you have glaucoma or if you're an alcoholic. Also, before giving Ludiomil,

COMPLICATING MEDICAL PROBLEMS

Before taking cyclic antidepressants, be sure to tell your doctor if you have any of the following medical problems:

➤ Alcohol abuse (cyclics may increase depressant effects of alcohol)
➤ Allergies (to cyclics, to maprotiline or trazodone, foods, preservatives, dyes)
➤ Asthma
➤ Blood disorders
➤ Contact lenses
➤ Convulsions or seizures
➤ Glaucoma or increased eye pressure
➤ Heart disease
➤ High blood pressure
➤ Intestinal problems (cyclics may cause increased risk of serious side effects)
➤ Kidney disease
➤ Liver disease (may raise blood levels of cyclics, causing more side effects)
➤ Manic depression
➤ Prostate enlargement
➤ Schizophrenia (cyclics may worsen schizophrenia)
➤ Stomach problems (cyclics may cause increased risk of serious side effects)
➤ Thyroid overactivity
➤ Urinary problems

your doctor will want to know if you have an enlarged prostate, stomach or intestinal problems, overactive thyroid, asthma, seizure disorders, or liver disease.

How to Use Cyclics

If your doctor is considering one of the cyclics to treat your depression, you may be asked to get a physical examination, an electrocardiogram (EKG), and routine blood tests first. These can help determine which type of drug will be safest for you to use.

No matter which cyclic you take, you'll begin with a small dose, gradually increasing in strength until your depression begins to improve. If you're one of those people who responds well to cyclics, you'll probably notice your sleeping problems improving within the first several days.

Some cyclics may work more quickly than others. A few people find that their depression disappears overnight—they go to sleep feeling depressed and wake up in a completely different mood. Others find their symptoms gradually fade over a period of days.

Don't get discouraged if you're not turning hand-springs within moments of starting therapy. Some people find it takes as long as three or four weeks before they see improvement.

Within a month, you'll probably notice that you're starting to be more interested in your surroundings, in other people and in activities that you once enjoyed. As the days pass, you should begin to feel better and better.

"When I began taking imipramine, I thought it would be like taking an aspirin—you pop it in and within an hour you feel different," says Carol. "It didn't happen that way. I began to feel gradual changes by the end of the second week, and by the third week there was quite a difference in my depression."

If you don't respond to a cyclic, it may mean your dose isn't high enough. Your doctor may order blood tests to find out how much of the drug is actually circulating in your blood, especially if you're taking imipramine, desipramine, nortriptyline, or amitriptyline. If after increasing the dose you still feel depressed after four or five weeks, your doctor will probably switch you to a different drug.

How Cyclics Are Administered

The usual adult dosage of protriptyline is 15 to 40 milligrams daily, divided into three or four doses. If necessary, doses may be increased up to 60 milligrams daily, but doses above this limit are not recommended. Any increases in amount should be given in the morning dose. Lower doses are recommended for adolescents and the elderly.

Your doctor will probably begin with about 75 milligrams of trimipramine daily in divided doses, increasing to 150 milligrams per day. Doses over 200 milligrams daily aren't recommended. Because this drug is so sedating, you can take the entire dose at bedtime.

Ludiomil may be taken in a single daily dose (usually at bedtime) or in divided daily doses. An initial dosage of 75 milligrams daily is usually effective. However, in some patients (such as the elderly, who tend to be oversensitive to antidepressants), an initial dose of 25 milligrams daily is recommended.

Because Ludiomil doesn't break down rapidly in the body, the initial dose should be maintained for at least two weeks. It may then be increased by 25-milligram increments as tolerated. Most people find that a maximum level of 150 milligrams is enough to keep symptoms under control. A maximum of 225 milligrams daily may be needed.

If you're taking Ludiomil for an extended period of time, your doctor may order blood cell counts and liver function studies and may monitor your blood pressure.

An overdose of a cyclic antidepressant may cause hallucinations, drowsiness, enlarged pupils, respiratory failure, fever, irregular heartbeat, severe dizziness, severe muscle

---

IF YOU FORGET A DOSE

ONE DAILY DOSE (BEDTIME)

➤ *Don't* take a missed bedtime dose in the morning, you may notice uncomfortable side effects during the day.

➤ Check with your doctor about getting back on the correct schedule.

MORE THAN ONE DAILY DOSE

➤ If you miss a dose, take the missed dose as soon as possible.

➤ If your missed dose is within an hour of the next one, skip the missed dose and get back on your regular dosage schedule.

➤ Don't double doses without your doctor's approval.

stiffness or weakness, restlessness or agitation, breathing problems, vomiting, convulsions, and coma. These drugs can be dangerous at fairly small amounts (10 to 15 times your normal dose)—and even smaller amounts in children.

Dietary Restrictions

There are some dietary cautions to keep in mind with specific cyclics. If you're taking the liquid version of doxepin (Adapin, Sinequan), don't mix it with grape juice or carbonated beverages, since these may reduce its effectiveness. Mix up this drug just before you take it.

Tolerance

While long-term treatment with antidepressants is controversial, more and more people are taking antidepressants for longer periods. Perhaps as a result, more and more of the antidepressants (even including some of the SSRIs, such as Prozac) are developing a reputation for decreasing effectiveness as treatment progresses.

This is known as tolerance, and among the tricyclics, amoxapine in particular has been associated with this problem. Once you develop tolerance to an antidepressant, you'll need higher doses in order to keep your depression under control.

Side Effects

On the whole, cyclics are pretty safe and effective, falling somewhere between the MAOIs, which have many side effects, and SSRIs, which have very few. Even if you do run into some unpleasant side effects in the beginning, chances are they will become less of a problem as time goes by. If not, you can always switch to a drug with a different side-effect profile.

Side effects with cyclics may include dry mouth, constipation, blurred vision, weight gain, increased heart rate, drowsiness, urinary retention, impotence, decreased blood pressure, and dizziness when standing up. Those with the highest probability for these side effects include amitriptyline, clomipramine, doxepin, imipramine and trimipramine. Desipramine has the lowest risk for these effects (see box: "Potential Side Effects with Cyclic Antidepressants"). And patients taking high doses of cyclics often complain of memory problems and trouble in finding the right words.

And like every other antidepressant, cyclics can trigger a mild manic high in some people. In a retrospective study published in the *British Medical Journal* of 3,065 patients with major depression, tricyclics worsened suicidal thinking slightly more than Prozac did (16.3 percent compared with 15.3 percent). Suicidal acts were reported as 0.3 percent for Prozac and 0.4 percent for tricyclics.

About 15 percent of people may feel nauseated (compared with about 21 percent of people taking Prozac); headaches occur in about 20 percent of people taking either Prozac or tricyclics.

Because some of these drugs are known for sedative effects that cause drowsiness, dizziness or decreased alertness, don't drive, fly an aircraft, operate dangerous machinery, or do anything requiring alertness until you learn how your medicine affects you. Following is a detailed explanation of the major cyclics' side effects:

POTENTIAL SIDE EFFECTS WITH CYCLIC ANTIDEPRESSANTS

COMMON SIDE EFFECTS

➤ Tremor   ➤ Headache

➤ Unpleasant taste   ➤ Sensitivity to sunlight

➤ Dry mouth   ➤ Constipation

➤ Nausea   ➤ Indigestion

➤ Fatigue   ➤ Insomnia

➤ Weakness   ➤ Sedation

➤ Anxiety   ➤ Nervousness

➤ Diarrhea   ➤ Excessive sweating

INFREQUENT ADVERSE EFFECTS

➤ Shakiness   ➤ Dizziness

➤ Vomiting   ➤ Abnormal dreams

➤ Eye pain   ➤ Diminished sex drive

➤ Slow pulse   ➤ Inflamed tongue

➤ Jaundice   ➤ Hair loss

➤ Joint Pain   ➤ Abdominal pain

➤ Palpitations   ➤ Fever

➤ Rash   ➤ Chills

➤ Palpitations   ➤ Visual changes

➤ Hiccups   ➤ Muscle aches

➤ Back pain   ➤ Nasal congestion

➤ Irregular heartbeat   ➤ Fainting

➤ Difficult and/or frequent urination

RARE ADVERSE EFFECTS

➤ Itchy skin   ➤ Sore throat

➤ Swollen testicles   ➤ Nightmares

continued

continued from previous page

➤ Swollen breasts   ➤ Confusion
➤ Involuntary movements of jaw, lips and tongue

SIDE EFFECTS MORE COMMON
TO PEOPLE OVER AGE 60
➤ Seizures   ➤ Hallucinations
➤ Headache   ➤ Shaking   ➤ Dizziness
➤ Fainting   ➤ Insomnia
➤ Urination problems

Dry mouth, blurred vision. As part of their action on many different brain systems, the cyclics act on histamine receptors, flicking on the body's "fight or flight" response, speeding up the heart, and shunting energy away from bodily functions, such as waste removal. The result: you get dry mouth, blurred vision, constipation, urinary problems. These side effects may be especially annoying if you're taking amitriptyline, clomipramine, doxepin, imipramine, or protriptyline.

"When I was taking imipramine, I had to chew gum all the time if I wanted to talk," remembers Gail, 52. "And I had to be sure I ate a jar of prunes every day—or else!" She notes that her dry mouth and constipation lasted for the entire two years she took imipramine.

If you're particularly bothered with a dry mouth, you can try sucking on sugarless candy or gum. (A lack of saliva can lead to tooth decay, so try not to aggravate this situation with sugar.) Or ask your physician to prescribe a saliva-promoting drug like pilocarpine.

Blood sugar levels. If you're a diabetic, you should be aware that cyclic antidepressants may affect your blood sugar levels. This means that you could notice your blood or urine test results are changing. If you have any questions, check with your doctor.

Constipation. It's important to remember that constipation may be a symptom of your depression and not a side effect of a cyclic antidepressant. If it is a symptom of your depression, the problem should disappear as the cyclic takes effect.

If it's clear you're constipated as a result of the drug, there are some dietary changes you can try. Begin by eating more fruits and vegetables, getting lots of fiber, and drinking plenty of fluids. If all other methods fail, your doctor can prescribe a stool softener or bulk agent. Finally, your doctor can switch you to an antidepressant that carries less of a risk for this type of side effect, such as Prozac or Zoloft or another of the newer antidepressants.

Contact lenses. You may experience problems with your contact lenses if you take cyclics. Because these drugs can cause dry eyes, your lenses may get gummed up with deposits of thick secretions, making them feel gritty, itchy, or painful. If this happens, your doctor may be able to prescribe a different antidepressant, reduce your dose, or prescribe artificial tears.

Dizziness. Some tricyclics, especially amitriptyline, might make you dizzy when you stand up (this is called "orthostatic hypotension"). If you notice this, try standing up more slowly. In the morning, dangle your feet over the side of the bed for a few minutes before slowly standing up. If you have a serious problem with dizziness, your doctor may be able to adjust your dose or switch you to another cyclic. The tricyclics least likely to cause this problem are amoxapine and nortriptyline (Pamelor).

Drowsiness. Sedation is a common side effect of many tricyclics and tetracyclics; three of the most sedating are doxepin, amitriptyline, and trimipramine.

"I found the sleepiness to be fairly pleasant," Sally, 52, reports. "I was sleepy all the time, but it was a blissful sort of sleepiness. And since I'd been having trouble sleeping before I started taking imipramine, I didn't mind it so much."

If you think that "drugged" feeling is unpleasant, you can try taking cyclics right before bedtime or ask your doctor about lowering your dosage. Or you may have more luck with one of the nonsedating tricyclics: amoxapine, desipramine (Norpramin, Pertofrane), nortriptyline, or protriptyline. These are a good choice if you experience lethargy and tiredness in addition to your depression. On the other hand, they may interfere with sleep, especially if you take your medication late in the day.

Neuroleptic malignant syndrome. If you use clomipramine too long, you run the small risk of developing a group of symptoms called "neuroleptic malignant syndrome," including fever, fast or irregular heartbeat, sweating, weakness, muscle stiffness, seizures, or loss of bladder control.

Sexual problems. Most antidepressants affect sexual functioning in one way or another, and cyclics aren't any different. You may experience either an increase or a decrease in sexual interest. Men may experience problems with erection or ejaculation or suffer from impotence. Cyclics may trigger swollen testicles, or breast enlargement in men and women. If you experience significant problems with sexual functioning, your doctor may choose to switch you to a different antidepressant that doesn't cause these problems, such as Wellbutrin (bupropion).

Sun sensitivity. If you take a cyclic antidepressant and you go out into the sun even briefly, you may end up with a rash, red or discolored skin, or a dreadful sunburn. Before

---

SUNLIGHT PRECAUTIONS
WHEN TAKING CYCLIC ANTIDEPRESSANTS

To prevent harmful skin reactions following exposure to sunlight, take the following precautions when you are taking cyclics:

➤ Stay out of direct sunlight between 10 A.M. and 3 P.M.

➤ If you have average skin, apply sun block with an SPF of at least 15; for fair or extremely sensitive skin, use a higher SPF number.

➤ Apply a lip sun-block with an SPF of at least 15.

➤ Wear protective clothing, a scarf or hat, and sunglasses.

➤ Do not use tanning booths or beds or sunlamps.

going out in the sun, study the accompanying list of "Sunlight Precautions When Taking Cyclic Antidepressants" (see box). If you do get a severe reaction from the sun, consult your doctor.

Sweating. Doxepin may interfere with sweating, making it harder for your body to withstand heat. To avoid the risk of heat stroke, avoid saunas or extremely hot climates while taking this drug.

Tardive dyskinesia. Amoxapine carries the risk of a group of unique side effects called "tardive dyskinesia"— speech or swallowing problems, lip smacking or puckering, loss of balance, cheek puffing, rapid or wormlike tongue movements, shakiness or trembling, shuffling walk, slow movements, arm or leg stiffness, uncontrolled chewing movements, and uncontrolled movements of hands, arms, or legs. This tardive dyskinesia may be permanent.

Weight gain. Many of the tricyclics cause weight gain. While it begins with just a few pounds, long-term treatment can add more and more weight until people stop taking the antidepressant (one study found that 48 percent of people stopped taking tricyclics because of weight gain). While there aren't any specific restrictions on diet, you may want to guard against eating too much to avoid gaining too much weight. You can take clomipramine with meals or after eating to lessen stomach distress.

If you're having a serious problem with weight gain, your doctor may want to consider one of the newer antidepressants (such as Wellbutrin, Paxil, Prozac, Zoloft, Desyrel, or Effexor), which don't usually cause weight gain.

Drug Interactions

Some medicines should never be used with cyclics (see box: "Potential Drug Interactions with Cyclic Antidepressants"), but other drug combinations are okay as long as your doctor monitors your condition closely.

Of course you'll want to avoid alcohol, which can be toxic when combined with cyclics. Taking cocaine with cyclics may cause irregular heartbeat; smoking marijuana may make you too sleepy. Some experts also believe that tobacco may make cyclics less effective.

There are also some specific interactions with a few of the cyclics. If you're taking desipramine, you should know that the effects of estrogen or birth-control pills may decrease the antidepressant's effectiveness.

Lithium will decrease the effectiveness of imipramine; imipramine's effects will be strengthened by simultaneously taking Prozac, estrogens, Ritalin, or birth-control pills. In addition, this drug may mask poisoning by organophosphorous-type insecticides.

Ludiomil may increase the effect of anticoagulants and may decrease the effect of guanethidine. Increased sedation may result by combining Ludiomil and anticholinergics or central-nervous-system depressants. The affects of Ludiomil may be increased if taken with cimetidine, thiazide, or Prozac, and may be decreased if taken with clonidine. Toxic symptoms may follow a combination of Ludiomil with methylphenidate. Finally, Ludiomil combined with levodopa may increase blood pressure.

The effects of clomipramine may be increased if taken with Prozac, Haldol, some diuretics, and Tagamet.

POTENTIAL DRUG INTERACTIONS
WITH CYCLIC ANTIDEPRESSANTS

- Alcohol
- Amphetamines (dextroamphetamine, methamphetamine)
- Anesthetics (plus some dental anesthetics)
- Aldomet
- Anticonvulsants (diazepam, phenobarbital, phenytoin, valproic acid, etc.)
- Antihistamine (Actifed, Benadryl, Chlor-Trimeton, Compoz, Dimetapp-DM)
- Appetite suppressants (fenfluramine, Preludin, Trimcaps, etc.)
- Barbiturates (Amytal, Nembutal, phenobarbital, Seconal, talbutal, etc.)
- Benzodiazepines (Dalmane, diazepam, Halcion, Librium, Valium, Xanax, etc.)
- Blood thinners (Coumadin, dicumarol, warfarin, etc.)
- Catapres
- Cylert
- Ephedrine (Broncholate, Ephed II, etc.)
- Hylorel
- Ismelin
- Isuprel
- MAOIs
- Muscle relaxants (cyclobenzaprine, dantrolene, orphenadrine, etc.)
- Neo-Synephrine
- Orap
- Phenergan
- Serpasil
- Sinus medication (Sinutab, Advil Sinus, etc.)
- Tagamet
- Temaril
- Tranquilizers (buspirone, chlorpromazine, haloperidol, thiothixene, etc.)
- Wellbutrin

If taken with Dilantin, chloral hydrate, or lithium, its effects may be decreased.

The effects of desipramine may be increased if taken with phenothiazine and decreased if taken with chloral hydrate, estrogen, lithium, or birth-control pills.

Imipramine's effects may be increased by taking it simultaneously with Tagamet, Prozac, or Ritalin. Its effects may be decreased by taking chloral hydrate or lithium at the same time.

Nortriptyline increases the effects of dicumarol and the drug's effects may be increased if taken with Tagamet or quinidine.

Pregnancy and Breast-feeding

If you're pregnant and seriously depressed, you and your doctor will have to weigh the risks of your untreated depression against possible damage to your fetus. While one study published in the January 1997 issue of *The New England Journal of Medicine* concluded that Prozac was safe to use during pregnancy, more research is needed.

Theoretically, all cyclics can pass into breast milk; therefore, you may want to discuss the wisdom of breast-feeding with your doctor if you are going to take cyclics after giving birth. The only specific negative information about tricyclics and breast-feeding infants is that doxepine may cause drowsiness in nursing babies.

Cyclics and Children

Imipramine is the most widely studied antidepressant when it comes to treating children. Because it's also one of the least toxic, it's the antidepressant most likely to be prescribed for youngsters. When a child is taking imipramine, his blood pressure, pulse, and heart rhythm should be monitored, since there's a greater risk of heart problems in youngsters between 6 and 12 than there is in adults. Despite extensive studies with children, no one knows whether this drug is safe for youngsters under age 6.

Imipramine is usually started at low doses (usually 25 milligrams daily) and increased by increments of 25 milligrams every few days until the depression begins to fade. Doses should always be given by an adult, since overdoses in children have been reported. Overdoses of tricyclics are particularly serious in children, who are unusually sensitive to these drugs. Doses should not exceed 2.5 milligrams per kilogram per day in children.

Because children are especially sensitive to all cyclics, they are at greater risk for side effects, especially nervousness, sleeping problems, fatigue, and mild stomach irritation. Check with your doctor if your child has any of these symptoms.

Cyclics and the Elderly

If you're over age 60 and take cyclics, don't be surprised if you experience one or more of these symptoms: confusion, dizziness, drowsiness, dry mouth, shakiness, fainting, constipation, urinary problems, headache, insomnia, and vision problems. Call your physician immediately if you experience any of these symptoms after you *stop* taking the drugs.

Cyclics and Obssessive-Compulsive Disorder

Antidepressants are sometimes used for other disorders besides depression, including obsessive-compulsive disorder, panic disorder, and (in the case of imipramine) bed-wetting.

As we learned in chapter 3, people with OCD become obsessed with certain thoughts and are bogged down with repetitive activities like washing themselves or rechecking doors and windows. The standard treatment for this disorder, which affects about 5 million Americans, is the tricyclic clomipramine, although in 1994 the FDA approved the SSRIs Prozac and Luvox as OCD treatments as well.

Because clomipramine must sometimes be taken in high doses (200 to 300 milligrams daily) to be effective against OCD, severe side effects are common. This is why more and more physicians are turning to Prozac, which produces only very mild side effects with this group.

Withdrawal

Once you and your doctor decide it's time for you to stop taking cyclics, don't just throw out the bottle and go on your way. First of all, you'll need to be careful not to stop taking your medication too soon, because your depression might return with renewed force. And there could also be some unpleasant consequences to an abrupt withdrawal from these antidepressants.

Most doctors advise their patients to take cyclics from six months to a year for best results. Others take antidepressants for much longer without apparent ill effects.

"With my doctor's okay, I've cut down my dosage of imipramine from 350 milligrams a day to 150," reports Carol. "My doctor tells me it's up to me as to how I feel. Eventually, I hope I can stop altogether. But if I feel a problem coming on, I'll go back on imipramine to keep from being depressed." You'll need to slowly decrease the dose if you've taken a cyclic for a long time, in order to lessen the risk of headaches, nausea, and overall discomfort.

The specter of side effects won't disappear after you stop taking the drug, however. You need to be aware that with this particular group of antidepressants, there are some side effects that may crop up only *after* you stop taking them. Check with your doctor if you notice any of the following: headache, irritability, lip smacking or puckering, nausea or vomiting, diarrhea, abdominal pain, convulsions, puffing of cheeks or rapid wormlike tongue movements, restlessness, insomnia, vivid dreams, uncontrolled chewing movements, uncontrolled leg or arm movements, or unusual excitement.

And remember, the medicine's effects may last up to seven days after you've stopped taking the pills. Observe all precautions about drug interactions and sun exposure listed in this chapter until a week after your treatment has stopped.

Conclusion

This chapter has described the creation of the very first antidepressants—and how they're still being used successfully by many people today. The next chapter will continue the antidepressant evolution, introducing the monoamine oxidase inhibitors—MAOIs.

6

Monoamine Oxidase Inhibitors

"MAO inhibitors worked much better for me than tricyclics. But for a chocoholic, the dietary restrictions were torture. That's why I finally stopped taking them."

—Marie, 42

Soon after scientists developed tricyclic antidepressants, another group of chemicals very different from the tricyclics rolled out of the laboratory—the monoamine oxidase (MAO) inhibitors. These new drugs affected the same neurotransmitters (serotonin and norepinephrine) that the tricyclics did, but they also affected dopamine.

How They Work

Once the brain's three neurotransmitters, known as monoamines (serotonin, norepinephrine, and dopamine), have played their part in sending messages in the brain, they get burned up by a protein in the brain called monoamine oxidase, a liver and brain enzyme.

Antidepressants known as monoamine oxidase inhibitors work by blocking this cleanup activity. When the excess neurotransmitters don't get destroyed, they start piling up in the brain. And since depression is associated with low levels of these monoamines, it's not surprising that *increasing* the monoamines ease depressive symptoms.

Unfortunately, monoamine oxidase doesn't just destroy those neurotransmitters; it's also responsible for mopping up another amine called tyramine, a molecule that affects blood pressure. So when monoamine oxidase

---

TYPES OF MAO INHIBITORS
AND THEIR DOSAGES

MAO INHIBITOR
isocarboxazid (Marplan)

    Usual Starting Dose: 30 mg/day

    Maximum Dose: 30 mg/day

phenelzine (Nardil)

    Usual Starting Dose: 15 mg/day

    Maximum Dose: 60 mg/day

tranylcypromine (Parnate)

    Usual Starting Dose: 30 mg/day

    Maximum Dose: 60 mg/day

gets blocked, levels of tyramine begin to rise, too. And that's when the trouble starts.

While a hike in neurotransmitters is beneficial, an increase in tyramine is disastrous. Excess tyramine can cause a sudden, sometimes fatal increase in blood pressure so severe that it can burst blood vessels in the brain.

Every time you eat chicken liver, aged cheese, broadbean pods, or pickled herring, tyramine floods into your brain. Normally, MAO enzymes take care of this potentially harmful tyramine excess. But if you're taking an MAO inhibitor, the MAO enzyme can't stop tyramine from building up. This is exactly what happened when the drugs were introduced in the 1960s. Because no one knew about the tyramine connection, a wave of deaths from brain hemorrhages swept the country. Other patients taking MAO inhibitors experienced severe headaches caused by the rise in blood pressure. These early side effects were particularly disturbing because nobody knew why they were happening.

The mystery was solved when a British pharmacist noticed that his wife, who was taking MAO inhibitors, got headaches when she ate cheese. But the early MAOIs were considered so dangerous (they also can damage the liver, brain, and cardiovascular systems) that even after the MAO-tyramine connection was finally understood, these drugs were taken off the American market for a time. (A related European antidepressant drug, Deprenyl, is marketed in this country as an anti-Parkinson's medication; it requires less stringent dietary cautions.)

Eventually the MAOIs were reintroduced in this country despite the tyramine risk because some depressed people don't respond to any other medication. Nevertheless, MAO inhibitors are usually the antidepressant of last resort.

"I call it the 'St. Jude' drug," says psychiatrist Andy Myerson. "It's the drug I use when nothing else works and someone is willing to give up anything in the hope that something will help their depression."

Prime Candidates

If you're very vulnerable to depression but don't suffer from the classic symptoms of major depression, MAOIs could be for you. They are especially good if you seem mildly depressed, if you become depressed more gradually, or if your primary complaints are boredom and apathy. If you have atypical depression—you're sensitive to rejection, overeat and oversleep, and react strongly to your environment—you may respond very well to MAOIs, which can reduce the sensitivity that causes you to feel so easily hurt or rejected. Others who tend to respond very well to MAOIs can feel quite depressed, but they're able to surface from the morass of their depression from time to time and experience pleasure before plunging into depression again.

The MAOI phenelzine (Nardil) has been found specifically to help patients characterized as atypical. These patients often have mixed anxiety and depression, or depression with phobia or hypochondriacal features. There is less evidence that Nardil may be effective in severely depressed patients. Tranylcypromine (Parnate) is a good choice if you have major depression without melancholia.

Who Shouldn't Take MAOIs

If you've got serious heart problems, epilepsy, bronchitis, asthma, or high blood pressure, or if you resist following a stringent diet, MAOIs aren't for you. In addition, isocarboxazid (Marplan) may be too stimulating if you're hyperactive, agitated, or schizophrenic. Studies suggest that Nardil may not be as effective if you are severely depressed. Patients should wait at least two weeks when being transferred to Parnate from another MAO inhibitor.

Pros and Cons

One of the big problems with MAO inhibitors is that they make you feel drugged and sluggish. "I didn't respond to tricyclics at all five years ago," says Karen, a New Jersey graduate student who has been chronically depressed most of her life. "When I was switched to an MAOI, I responded very well. But I couldn't take the diet. After I finally went off the drug, my friends told me I was always in a daze while I was taking MAOIs, but I wasn't aware of that at the time. I was switched to Prozac four years ago, and I've been taking that ever since." Patients often look dazed or even robotic, much the way Karen had appeared to her friends. But what people really hate are the lists of dietary restrictions and potential side effects.

"A lot of patients are resentful about the diet they have to follow," explains Dr. Myerson. "They tend to blame the doctor when they can't eat their favorite foods, and many people simply won't follow the diet." Other mental health experts point out that MAO inhibitors often interfere with the relationship between doctor and patient, because people feel so resentful about their side effects and diet that they don't want to talk to their doctor during therapy.

DIETARY RESTRICTIONS

Don't eat or drink any of the following when taking MAOIs unless your doctor advises otherwise:

Aged foods
Alcoholic beverages (especially Chianti, sherry, liqueurs, and beer)
Alcohol-free or reduced-alcohol beer or wine
Anchovies
Bologna, pepperoni, salami, summer sausage, or any fermented sausage
Caviar
Cheeses (especially strong or aged varieties), except for cottage and cream cheese
Chicken livers
Fermented foods
Figs (canned)
Fruit: raisins, bananas (or any overripe fruit)
Meat prepared with tenderizers; unfresh meat; meat extracts
Smoked or pickled meat, poultry, or fish
Soy sauce

Foods you can eat in moderation:

Avocados
Beer
Caffeine (including chocolate, coffee, tea, cola)
Chocolate
Raspberries
Sauerkraut
Soup (canned or powdered)
Sour cream
Yogurt

Their relatively risky profile makes them a poor choice for potentially suicidal patients who might intentionally take an overdose. At very low doses, the MAOIs can have toxic effects on the heart, unlike Prozac, which is not considered toxic even at very high doses. Studies have shown that MAOIs are not associated *at all* with suicide in nonsuicidal patients, as opposed to most other antidepressants. In a 1991 Harvard University study of 1,017 depressed people, 63 nonsuicidal patients took an MAOI and none became suicidal.

On the other hand, there's no doubt that for a certain subset of people, the MAO inhibitors work better than any other antidepressant.

"I've seen a few miracle cures with these drugs," one psychiatrist noted. "And they're particularly good if people suffer from panic attacks in addition to depression."

Furthermore, if you have hypertension or heart problems, the MAOIs might be for you because at therapeutic doses, they can *lower* blood pressure. In contrast to the tricyclic antidepressants, MAO inhibitors have little negative effect on heart rate.

If you were having problems with chest pain (angina) before taking MAO inhibitors, you may find that you're feeling much better now that you're taking this drug. Whatever you do, don't start running a few extra miles or working out a lot more at the gym without first discussing it with your doctor! Too much activity can bring on another attack of chest pain.

Before Taking MAOIs

Your doctor will probably quiz you about a range of medical conditions before prescribing an MAO inhibitor. *It's especially important to tell your doctor if you have frequent headaches or chest pain.* Since a severe headache or chest pain during MAOI therapy is the primary warning sign of a serious spike in blood pressure, anyone who *normally* gets severe headaches might overlook an important warning sign.

Your doctor will want to know if you have diabetes mellitus (you may need to change your insulin level) or an alcohol problem, since drinking while taking MAOIs may cause serious side effects.

Also tell your doctor if you have heart or blood-vessel disease, liver or kidney problems, Parkinson's disease, or an overactive thyroid.

Side Effects

The one thing you've got to watch out for with these drugs is that sudden spike in blood pressure called a "hypertensive crisis" (also called the "cheese reaction") that we discussed at the beginning of this chapter. As long as you follow a strict tyramine-free diet (see box: "Dietary Restrictions"), you should be able to avoid the risk.

Diet-Related Side Effects. Your doctor most assuredly will give you a list of prohibited foods. It's important to remember that the tyramine found in foods—even a type of food that can be eaten in small quantities—adds up. So while it's okay to eat small amounts of sour cream or artichokes, it would not be acceptable to eat a meal of sauerkraut with a sauce of yogurt and sour cream, followed by a dessert of raspberries and chocolate together with a cup of coffee.

It's also important to understand that while you may get away with eating a forbidden food once or twice, it may cause a reaction the third or fourth time. This is because a particular food doesn't always contain the same amount of tyramine.

The symptoms are as follows: severe headache radiating to the front of the head, stiff and/or sore neck, nausea and vomiting, sensitivity to light, dilated pupils, sweating (sometimes with fever or with cold, clammy skin), chest pain, or heart palpitations. A blood pressure rise usually occurs within several hours after taking the drug. *Stop taking MAO inhibitors immediately if you get a severe headache or palpitations,* then call your doctor.

Your doctor can give you a drug called Procardia as an emergency measure if you accidentally eat something that causes a reaction.

There is also a range of less serious side effects that accompany the MAOIs. Like all antidepressants, the MAOIs are capable of inducing a manic state in people who are manic-depressive. Like tricyclics, MAOIs have been reported to cause memory problems. Other possible side effects include:

Fainting and/or Dizziness. If you're taking an MAOI, you may feel a bit dizzy or faint if you stand up quickly. It's a common side effect with these drugs and is more annoying than anything else. It can lead to giddiness, muscular weakness, nausea, perspiration, hyperventilation,

GENERAL SIDE EFFECTS OF ALL **MAO** INHIBITORS

Stop taking this drug and seek immediate help for:

Unusually high blood pressure

Severe chest pain	Fast or slow heartbeat
Severe headache	Increased sensitivity to light
Increased sweating	Nausea and vomiting
Stiff or sore neck	

Check with your doctor if you have:

Severe dizziness or light-headedness, especially when arising from a sitting or lying position

Diarrhea	Pounding heartbeat

Swelling of feet and/or lower legs

Unusual excitement or nervousness

Dark urine	Fever
Skin rash	Slurred speech
Sore throat	Staggering walk

Yellow eyes and/or skin

Mild side effects not usually requiring medical attention:

Blurry vision	Decreased sexual ability
Urinary problems	Drowsiness
Mild headache	Weight gain
Increased sweating	Restlessness
Shakiness or trembling	Fatigue and weakness
Sleeping problems	Chills
Constipation	Decreased appetite
Dry mouth	Muscle twitching during sleep

Increased appetite (especially for sweets) and mild dizziness or light-headedness and sometimes confusion. If this happens to you, try standing up more slowly. (You may notice that you have a particular problem when you get up in the morning; this is because blood pressure is lowest then. If this happens, sit on the edge of the bed, dangling your feet for a minute or two, and then rise slowly.)

This problem often fades away with time. If it doesn't, you can try exercising your leg muscles to prevent blood from pooling in your legs. It may also help to wear support hosiery and drink plenty of fluids.

If the problem gets worse, ask your doctor if you can divide your medication into several doses to be taken during the day. Try taking the medicine after meals, and take salt tablets.

Drowsiness. Because MAO inhibitors may cause blurred vision, drowsiness, or a "drugged" feeling, be sure you know how you react to this medicine before you do anything that could be dangerous if your alertness or vision were affected, such as driving or operating machinery.

Diabetes. If you're a diabetic, MAO inhibitors may affect your blood sugar levels. While using these antidepressants, be very careful when you're testing the sugar levels in your blood or urine. Consult with your doctor if you have any questions about your diabetic condition.

Sexual Problems. Like many other antidepressants, MAOIs can cause a range of sexual problems. Of these, delayed orgasm is the most common (it is also very likely with Prozac). However, many people note that sexual problems eventually disappear.

Surgery. Be sure to tell your doctor or dentist that you're taking MAO inhibitors before any kind of surgery, dental treatment or emergency treatment—even if you stopped taking the drug up to two weeks ago. The anesthesia combined with the MAOIs can cause a drop in blood pressure or other problems. You may want to carry an ID card noting that you're taking this medicine. If you're taking these drugs, you shouldn't agree to any elective surgery requiring general anesthesia.

Weight Gain. MAOIs are associated with some degree of weight gain. (Prozac and some other SSRIs do not seem to cause this side effect.)

Drug Interactions

While aspirin, Tylenol (plain), Motrin, or antibiotics are safe when combined with MAOIs, you should check with your doctor before taking *any other medicine.*

There have been reports of serious—sometimes fatal—reactions when an MAO inhibitor is combined with Prozac. These reactions include high blood pressure, nausea and vomiting, fever, rigidity, rapidly fluctuating vital signs, shock, and mental changes. You shouldn't take Prozac until two weeks after stopping therapy with an MAO inhibitor. Even more important, because Prozac takes a long time to be eliminated from the body, *you should wait at least five weeks after stopping Prozac before you start taking an MAO inhibitor.*

Besides Prozac, there are some other medications that can provoke a hypertensive reaction similar to the cheese reaction (but not involving tyramine). Of these, the most dangerous are nonprescription cold, cough, or sinus medications such as Contac or Dristan; most of them contain decongestants (like pseudoephedrine). Other drugs on the danger list include weight-control pills and asthma inhalants. Illegal drugs like cocaine and amphetamines also cause this problem.

Most of the medications that cause problems are stimulants that can trigger an increase in the release of norepinephrine, which raises blood pressure. Since MAO metabolizes norepinephrine, people taking MAOIs have higher amounts of norepinephrine to be released, which raises the blood level of norepinephrine even more.

The opiate narcotics Demerol (meperidine) and dextromethorphan (found in cough or cold medicines usually labeled "DM") should also be avoided. And Parnate can interfere with the benefit of guanethidine, methyldopa, reserpine, and dopamine. Nardil shouldn't be taken with dopamine, epinephrine and norepinephrine, methyldopa, L-dopa, L-tryptophan, L-tyrosine or phenylalanine (contained in aspartame, also known as NutraSweet).

Overdose

The MAO inhibitors are somewhat more dangerous drugs than other antidepressants when taken in excessive amounts—far more so than newer drugs such as Prozac, Zoloft or Desyrel. Symptoms of overdose include severe anxiety, confusion, convulsions or seizures, cool clammy skin, severe dizziness, severe drowsiness, fast and irregular pulse, fever, hallucinations, severe headache, high or low blood pressure, muscle stiffness, breathing problems, severe sleeping problems, or unusual irritability.

DRUG INTERACTIONS AND MAO INHIBITORS

Some drugs should never be combined with MAO inhibitors, while others may be used if your doctor adjusts your dosage. It's extremely important for you to tell your doctor if you are taking any of the following drugs:

Allergy medicines (including nose drops or sprays)
Appetite suppressants
Antihistamines (Actifed DM, Benadryl, Benylin, Chlor-Trimeton, Compoz, etc.)
Antipsychotics
Antivert
Asthma drugs
Atrovent
Blood-pressure medicine
Bucladin
BuSpar (may cause high blood pressure)
Cocaine (may severely increase blood pressure)
Cold medicines
Demerol (deaths have occurred when combining MAOIs and a single dose of meperidine)
Dextromethorphan (may cause brief episodes of psychosis or bizarre behavior)
Ditropan
Dopar, Larodopa
Flexeril
Insulin (MAOIs may change amount of insulin needed)
Ludiomil
Marezine

Monoamine oxidase inhibitors (other)
Norflex
Norpace
Phenergan
Pronestyl
Prozac (may cause high fever, rigidity, high blood
    pressure, mental changes, confusion and hypoma-
    nia; at least five weeks should pass between stop-
    ping Prozac and starting an MAOI)
Quinidex
Ritalin
Sinus medicine
Symmetrel
Tegretol (may increase seizures)
Temaril (may increase chance of side effects)
Tricyclic antidepressants (using these drugs within two
    weeks of taking MAOIs may cause serious side
    effects including sudden fever, extremely high
    blood pressure, convulsions, and death)
Tryptophan (may cause disorientation, confusion,
    amnesia, delirium agitation, hypomanic signs, shiv-
    ering)
Urispas
Wellbutrin (allow at least two weeks between stopping
    Wellbutrin and starting MAOIs)

Tolerance

Some people develop a tolerance to MAO inhibitors. This
could mean that the drug will work for you at first, but
you could suddenly become depressed again in the middle
of treatment. This sort of reaction is particularly disturbing because it sets off a plummeting depression that may
not respond to any other antidepressant. Oddly, if you

develop tolerance to an MAOI, the best solution may be to switch to another antidepressant for a few weeks, and then start taking the same MAOI again. This way, the drug may regain its effectiveness.

Withdrawal

Don't suddenly stop taking this medicine on your own. Your doctor will probably ask you to gradually taper off your dosage to avoid the risk of side effects. Once you do stop taking the drug, remember that you must continue to observe all of the dietary restrictions *for at least two weeks*, avoiding all of the same foods and beverages that you did when you were taking MAO inhibitors.

Pregnancy and/or Breast-feeding

Because Parnate (and most likely Marplan and Nardil) cross the placenta, you and your doctor should weigh the need for this drug against the risks to your unborn child. Nardil has been shown to have adverse effects in pregnant mice; in doses well above the human dose it has caused decreases in the number of healthy offspring. While researchers don't know for sure whether antidepressants cause birth defects in humans, women who take any type of antidepressant have about twice the rate of miscarriages during the first trimester of pregnancy. As with most anti-depressants, safe use of MAO inhibitors during pregnancy hasn't been established, but one limited study in humans did suggest an increased risk of birth defects when MAOIs are taken during the first trimester.

In animals, MAO inhibitors slow the growth of new-borns and make them more excitable when their mothers take very large doses during pregnancy.

When it comes to breast-feeding, Parnate is passed into breast milk, but it is not known if this is true of Marplan and Nardil. There haven't been any reports of problems in nursing infants whose mothers have taken MAO inhibitors.

MAOIs and Children

Because MAOIs are among the most risky of antidepressants, most experts don't recommend giving them to children under age 16. Animal studies indicate that these drugs may slow growth in the young.

MAOIs and the Elderly

Older patients are usually more sensitive than younger adults to the MAO inhibitors, and they may be more likely to experience dizziness or light-headedness. Because of the danger of an abrupt increase in high blood pressure (hypertensive crisis), the MAO inhibitors are often not prescribed for people over age 60, or for those with heart or blood-vessel diseases.

Parnate should not be routinely given to anyone over age 60 because of the possibility of damaged blood vessels and the risk of sudden high blood pressure; you should wait at least two weeks before being transferred from Parnate to another MAOI. In this event, the starting dose should be half the normal starting dose for the first week of therapy.

Other Uses

MAOIs have been shown to be effective in the treatment of a wide range of disorders besides depression. They are very good at treating eating disorders—but the weight gain they often cause can be counterproductive. Prozac, on the other hand, is just as effective as an eating-disorder treatment, without the unwanted side effects. In one recent study of 400 women, Prozac cut down on eating binges in 63 percent of the responders and vomiting in up to 57 percent.

For social phobics, for whom the idea of a social occasion can produce a range of negative emotions and symptoms, MAOIs (especially Nardil) can be very helpful. In fact, studies suggest that about 70 percent of people who are social phobics respond to MAOIs. Recent research has also suggested that Prozac may also be effective for this problem.

MAOIs are also helpful in treating panic disorder, social phobia, agoraphobia, obsessive-compulsive disorder, and attention-deficit disorder.

Conclusion

You've seen how difficult the MAOIs can be, and how helpful they are to a subgroup of people who respond well to them. In the next chapter, we'll learn about a group of maverick drugs that are structurally unlike any other class of antidepressants—Wellbutrin, Desyrel and Effexor.

7

STRUCTURALLY
UNRELATED DRUGS

---

*"When I was depressed, it was like having a tight
metal band around my head all the time. I felt like
my cognitive processes couldn't run with the energy
they should have. When I took Wellbutrin and my
depression lifted, the band loosened and the relief
was incredible."*

—*Jim, 42*

Jim was the son of two alcoholics, a brilliant but erratic
man who blazed through his adolescence and early
adulthood and crashed into a fog of depression in medical
school. For the next 10 years, he was haunted by inter-
mittent episodes of depression. But it was his inability to
function at work that Jim, a drug company executive,
found most troubling.

"The problems my depression was causing me at
work were particularly devastating," he recalls today. "I
was trying to build my ego late in life, which is fairly
common among children of alcoholics. And my depression was getting in the way of my healthy functioning."

In a vain attempt at self-medication, Jim began using cocaine regularly. When he was finally given a prescription for Wellbutrin, he had given up hope that he would ever regain his ability to think clearly.

Within a week, he began to notice an effect. Within five or six weeks, his depression was gone. "Being able to focus again on work, instead of on myself and my problems, was initially the most uplifting effect," he recalls. Wellbutrin also helped him overcome his cocaine addiction.

Bupropion (Wellbutrin), trazodone (Desyrel), venlafaxine (Effexor), and mirtazapine (Remeron) are a group of structurally unrelated antidepressants that don't fit into any of the established antidepressant drug classes of MAOIs, tricyclics, or SSRIs.

These three are among a group of drugs that scientists have discovered as a result of fiddling with the biochemistry of antidepressants, looking for the perfect medication that's safe, nontoxic, and effective. Although all three are very effective antidepressants, each one affects a different neurotransmitter system: Wellbutrin affects dopamine, Desyrel affects serotonin, and Effexor affects norepinephrine, serotonin, and dopamine, while Remeron stimulates norepinephrine and serotonin release as it blocks certain receptors.

Pros and Cons

Wellbutrin, Effexor, Desyrel, and Remeron appear to cause fewer serious side effects than MAO inhibitors or tricyclics. But because these three drugs can cause a few unusual problems in some people, chances are your psychiatrist will be far more likely to choose an SSRI like Prozac or Zoloft at first.

The most common side effects shared by Wellbutrin, Effexor, and Desyrel include agitation, dry mouth, insomnia, headache, nausea and vomiting, constipation, and tremors.

But perhaps the most troubling problem with the newer drugs is that no one is sure just what their long-term effects might be. There are some new, troubling reports that Effexor may cause tardive dyskinesia, a movement disorder that may be permanent, involving writhing, wormlike movements of the body, lips, and tongue.

But many chronically depressed people say they don't care. They're willing to pay the price of future uncertainty to buy freedom from depression today.

"There are risks to these drugs," says Joan, whose training as a nurse makes her more aware than most of the possible hazards. "They just don't know what they do in the body. But after this many years of being depressed, it's worth the risk to me. I've spent half my life in hell, so taking a risk with antidepressants is well worth the effort. As more years have gone by, I see the years I was depressed as wasted. I don't want to waste any more."

Wellbutrin

The good news about Wellbutrin is that you probably won't have sexual problems, you won't gain weight (you may even lose a few pounds!), and you won't have a lot of annoying minor side effects. The bad news is that—especially if you've had a head injury or you have epilepsy—there's a higher risk of seizures.

"Wellbutrin is usually my second-choice antidepressant," says psychiatrist Andy Myerson. "I've had remarkable success with it, but many people are scared by the potential for seizures. It's tricky."

Because Wellbutrin blocks dopamine, this drug also can rarely produce movement disorders and changes in the endocrine system.

As mentioned above, the biggest problem associated with Wellbutrin is the fact that psychiatrists are nervous about a risk of seizure four times higher than with other antidepressants. Overdosing is a particular danger, since the chance of a seizure increases almost tenfold at twice the normal daily dose of 300 milligrams. Your biggest chance of developing a seizure appears to be if you've had a prior serious head injury or prior seizures, brain or spinal-cord tumors, if you take anti-seizure medication, or if you suddenly hike your dosage. You can lower the risk if you never abruptly increase your dosage, don't take more than 450 milligrams a day, and limit any single dose to no more than 150 milligrams.

Some patients find that Wellbutrin's action on the central nervous system can produce unpleasant hypersensitivity. "When I took Wellbutrin, I spent a lot of time on my sofa with the blanket over my head," comments Eleanor, 39, a Colorado stockbroker. "I felt oversensitized all over my body. I just felt weird."

But others have found benefit with the drug. Since Wellbutrin is not sedating, you feel some effect right away because you don't have to work your way through the haze of sedation produced by the tricyclics and MAOIs.

"I took tricyclics for about four days. I was so sleepy, my face fell into my food at Thanksgiving," recalls Jim.

"But with Wellbutrin, I was able to work again, and that gave me hope. Hope is something you don't have when you're depressed."

One of the most demoralizing problems with almost all antidepressants is their negative effect on sexual function, such as decreased libido, erection problems, and impotence. Wellbutrin's boost to the libido can come as a welcome relief to many people; indeed, some patients can find Wellbutrin too sexually stimulating.

"I was thinking about sex all the time," complains Hilary, 39, who was given Wellbutrin when Zoloft did not relieve her depression. "I spent all my time in bed."

While there have been no reports that Wellbutrin caused liver damage, animal studies have revealed a variety of liver problems with this drug. And don't be surprised if you feel restless; some number of people taking Wellbutrin report some amount of agitation, anxiety, and insomnia, especially at the beginning of treatment. Some people have needed to be treated with sedatives or hypnotic drugs to ease the anxiety. A new formulation of Wellbutrin, Wellbutrin SR, has a more favorable side effect profile than the original version.

"Psychiatrists end up getting the treatment failures from other people," says Dr. Myerson. "Almost everything causes sexual problems, and with Wellbutrin there is less of that. But when people don't like Wellbutrin, they *really* hate it."

Very rarely, patients treated with either Wellbutrin or Desyrel develop serious mental symptoms including delusions, hallucinations, psychotic episodes, confusion, paranoia, hostility, disorientation, memory problems, or nightmares, but studies have not shown what the exact percentage risk may be. In some cases, the symptoms decreased when the dosage was decreased or withdrawn.

Desyrel

Then there's Desyrel. Unlike antidepressants such as Prozac that may keep you pacing the floor at night, Desyrel can have you sleeping like a baby. On the down side, on rare occasions Desyrel may cause a nasty side effect called priapism, a painful erection of the penis without sexual arousal. Priapism occurs when blood doesn't drain from the penis's spongy tissue, keeping it erect. Urgent treatment is needed because of the risk of permanent damage to the penis. Other patients experience permanent impairment of erection or impotence.

Desyrel has also been linked to some heart problems, and birth defects in animals.

Some of the side effects of these drugs may actually work for you. For example, because of Desyrel's sedative qualities, it's often added to other drugs like Prozac, if insomnia becomes a problem.

"Before taking antidepressants, I was having a lot of trouble sleeping because of my depression," notes Sarah, 42. "After a few weeks on Prozac, I still wasn't sleeping, so my psychiatrist added Desyrel. I take it right before I go to sleep, and I've been sleeping again for the first time in years."

Remeron (mirtazapine)

Approved by the FDA in July 1996, Remeron offers another approach to the treatment of depression and is often helpful for people having trouble with sleep and anxiety. The first of a new class of drugs, Remeron does not broadly block the reuptake of norepinephrine or serotonin like other SSRIs. Instead, Remeron stimulates the release of norepinephrine and serotonin, while blocking certain receptors that have been linked with lowered sex drive, nausea, nervousness, headache, insomnia, and diarrhea. As a result, Remeron does not usually lead to any of these side effects. Many people have been particularly troubled by the loss of sexual interest or ability with SSRIs; but, in United States studies, a lowered sex drive occurred in only one percent of patients receiving Remeron.

This doesn't mean that Remeron is free of side effects. For some people, fatigue, weight gain, increased appetite, and dizziness can be troublesome. Still, the dropout rate is low; in U.S. studies only about 16 percent of patients stopped taking the drug because of unpleasant side effects.

"I didn't think I'd ever feel this good again," said Joe, a 43-year-old severely depressed teacher who had tried several other antidepressants without success. "I even got my sex life back!"

Caution: Anyone who is taking Remeron who develops an infection and has a low white-blood-cell count should stop the drug. It should be used with caution in those with liver or kidney problems. Older patients (especially older men) may find it takes longer for the drug to clear their system. As with SSRIs, you should not take Remeron at the same time as a monoamine oxidase inhibitor (MAOI) or use it within two weeks of stopping or starting MAOI treatment.

Effexor

If you had your heart set on taking Prozac and were disappointed when nothing happened, there's a drug that seems to work especially well for the up to 40 percent who don't respond to serotonin-related antidepressants. It's called Effexor, approved in 1994 by the FDA. Because Effexor is structurally unlike SSRIs, people who don't respond to Prozac, Zoloft, or one of the tricyclics often do respond to this antidepressant. It's so new, however, that doctors don't know a lot about how this drug will act on a long-term basis. As mentioned above, there are some concerns that this drug may cause tardive dyskinesia—usually after long-term use, although there have been some cases appearing after only one dose.

Tricia, 39, is a Boston nurse who ended up taking Effexor for a lifelong depression after trying every known tricyclic. "The first effects of Effexor were visual," she recalls. "I felt as if there was a cool breeze blowing behind my eyes. Colors were sharper, and all my senses perked up. I feel the way I imagine normal people feel, without struggling through the haze of depression. It clarified things."

The feeling of clarity was especially important to Tricia, who was terrified that the muted experience of her depression would lead her to make mistakes at work. "I was constantly afraid I would kill someone," she recalls. As a result, she became hypervigilant at work, putting so much energy into her job that at the end of the day she was totally exhausted.

"Before Effexor, every morning I would usually have a few suicidal thoughts before I left for work in the morning. Now I'm afraid that this (normal feeling) will be taken away."

Before Taking These Drugs

Just as with other antidepressants, you've got to be sure to tell your doctor if you've ever had allergies to any antide-pressants, foods, preservatives, or dyes, and if you have suf-fered from manic depression, convulsions, or seizures. Be sure to report liver disease, since this condition may raise blood levels of any antidepressant, which can in-crease the risk of side effects. If you have any type of seizure disorder, recent head injury, brain or spinal-cord tumor, bulimia, or anorexia nervosa, you shouldn't take Wellbutrin either, since all of these problems have been associated with a higher risk for seizures. And if you've had a recent heart attack, you may not be able to take antidepressant medication.

Additional Tests

If you're taking Wellbutrin, talk to your doctor about the possible need for follow-up medical exams or studies to check kidney and liver function or blood levels of the drug.

When taking Desyrel, you may need to take com-plete blood-cell-count tests, since this drug can reduce your white-blood-cell count. (White blood cells are an important part of your body's immune system, and low levels could be a problem if you develop an infection, sore throat, or fever.) Because of the link between Desyrel and some heart problems, your doctor may ask you to have blood-pressure readings and electrocardiograms.

How to Take These Drugs

To lessen stomach upset, it's a good idea to take any of these three drugs with meals unless your doctor has specifically asked you to take your medication on an empty stomach.

When taking Wellbutrin, you should equally divide your medication into three or four doses a day to minimize the risk of seizure. Never drink alcohol while taking Wellbutrin, since this also may increase the risk of seizure.

If you get too sleepy or dizzy with Desyrel, ask your doctor if you can take a larger portion of your total daily dose at bedtime, dividing the rest into two or three smaller doses during the day.

Possible Drug Interactions

As with all antidepressants, you should talk to your doctor before taking any other drugs (even nonprescription medications).

Taking Wellbutrin with a tricyclic antidepressant may increase the risk of seizure. Taking Wellbutrin with an MAO inhibitor, or within two weeks of taking an MAO inhibitor, will increase the chance of side effects. At least two weeks should pass between stopping one medication and taking another.

Overdose

An overdose is less of a problem with the newer antidepressants. That's another reason why doctors like to give these newer drugs to suicidal patients—they're less likely to be able to take a fatal overdose. If you overdose on

Wellbutrin, you'll probably recover, although you might experience seizures or hallucinations or lose consciousness. Still, there have been cases of heart failure and fatalities from Wellbutrin overdoses.

Pregnancy and Breast-feeding

If you want to get pregnant while you're on an antidepressant, you're going to have to weigh the risks to your baby against the risks to you if you *don't* take the drug. As with most antidepressants, what we know about their activity in pregnant women is mostly obtained from animal studies, not from large-scale studies in humans.

Your best choice might be Wellbutrin, which hasn't caused birth defects or other development problems in animal studies even in doses up to 45 times the human daily dose. The effect of Wellbutrin on labor and delivery in humans isn't known, however.

Desyrel seems a little more risky; animal studies with this drug have revealed fetal deaths and birth defects. As a result, use of Desyrel is not recommended during the first three months of pregnancy.

You and your doctor should weigh the potential risks to the fetus and to you before you decide whether or not to take antidepressants during pregnancy.

There's always a potential for adverse reactions in nursing infants (especially with Wellbutrin). If you're a new mom, you need to weigh the risks to you of not taking medication against the potential harm to your baby.

Use with the Elderly

If you're over age 60, you're more likely to be sensitive to all of the antidepressants. This means your depression will probably respond to lower doses of medication. It also means you are at higher risk for developing side effects.

Some antidepressants may be a better choice than others, of course. For example, studies with Wellbutrin in a limited number of patients over age 60 haven't found any problems caused by the drug.

Conclusion

In this chapter we've focused on four new drugs that are unrelated to each other or any of the earlier classes of anti-depressants. In the next chapter, we'll discuss lithium, a unique medication that's used specifically for one type of depression—that which occurs with bipolar disorder, or manic depression (the older term for bipolar disorder).

8

LITHIUM

"When I went off lithium, the manic depression came back. I was barely able to go to work. It was terrible. I would stand there at work and pretend I was alive."
—Jack, 48

Jack had been consumed with energy all his life, but in his early twenties experienced his first heavy depression. Diagnosed as a classic manic-depressive, he began taking lithium and was able to live a fairly normal life until 1989, when his doctors briefly stopped his lithium treatment.

During this period, Jack spiraled into a state he describes as "close to death," a depression so profound he didn't know whether he would survive. By the time he was put back on lithium, he no longer responded to the drug. Now considered to be "lithium resistant," he takes a combination of the antiepileptics Tegretol and Depakote, the drugs of choice for people who no longer respond to lithium.

For Jack, the combination "is only about 40 percent effective," he says. Jack is a "rapid cycler," with a mixed state of manic-depression. This means that instead of

---

LITHIUM TOXICITY SYMPTOMS

Remember: It's easy for toxic levels of lithium to build up if you have kidney problems or low salt levels, if you get dehydrated or take diuretics, or during childbirth.

<u>EARLY SIGNS</u>
➤ Diarrhea and vomiting
➤ Drowsiness
➤ Muscular weakness
➤ Lack of coordination

<u>HIGHER TOXICITY</u>
➤ Giddiness/confusion
➤ Blurred vision
➤ Tinnitus (ringing of the ears)
➤ Seizures
➤ Staggering gait

---

extended episodes of depression and then mania lasting for several months each, he cycles constantly through mania and depression. The drugs he takes don't eradicate this process, but they tone it down so that his lows aren't quite so devastating and his highs aren't quite so manic.

What Is Lithium?

Lithium is an element of the periodic table that readily forms salts. As early as 200 A.D., the Greek physician Galen was prescribing alkaline spring baths for manic patients.

Lithium *bromide* was used as a sedative beginning in the early 1900s, but it fell into disfavor in the 1940s when some heart patients died after using it as a salt substitute. Almost immediately thereafter, a little-known psychiatrist in Australia discovered that lithium salts were extremely effective in treating manic-depression.

Eventually, lithium's popularity grew, until by the late 1960s it was once again widely prescribed in this country, when it was heralded as the first effective treatment for manic depression.

Excreted by the kidneys, lithium carbonate has a narrow range between toxic and therapeutic doses. It's used mostly to manage manic-depression, to smooth out the hills and valleys of a person's emotional swings and the lows of chronic recurring depression. It can quickly reverse acute mania in 80 percent of people, and stabilize mood in 60 to 70 percent.

How Does It Work?

While scientists aren't quite sure how this drug works, they believe it may correct chemical imbalances in certain nerve impulse transmitters (serotonin and norepinephrine) that influence emotional status and behavior.

While lithium can have a mild antidepressant effect, it's primarily effective for its strong anti-manic effects, working best by controlling the highs of mania. If you're taking lithium to control manic highs but you're still depressed, your doctor may want to add Prozac or another antidepressant, which is helpful for long-term control of manic-depression.

Lithium can also be effective in the treatment of major depression, and can boost the effectiveness of tricyclics, MAOIs, or SSRIs when these drugs don't quite get the job done on their own.

Is Lithium for all Manic-Depressives?

Unfortunately, lithium doesn't work well for everyone; it's most effective for those who've had no more than three episodes of mania. About 20 percent of people will have a complete remission on lithium, and the rest will have varying degrees of relief. Some will experience fewer episodes of mania; those that do occur are shorter and less severe, and people feel more stable between manic episodes. But for some people, lithium may just stop working.

Unfortunately, lithium no longer works for Jack, whose partially uncontrolled manic-depression is so debilitating he can't work. In his depressed state, he can't concentrate, can't read, feels lethargic, and has memory problems. Then he'll suddenly shoot up into mania, with too much energy and a "horrible libido."

Jack's case is an example of a person with progressive manic-depression, whose disorder worsens over time; lithium can stop working for these people, and the alternatives (Tegretol and Depakote) may not be completely effective. Because some experts believe that progressive manic-depression is a result of structural changes in the brain as the disease worsens, they recommend keeping people on lithium for long periods of time to prevent the almost-impossible-to-reverse deterioration. (This theory is controversial.)

In about 30 percent of manic-depressives, lithium smooths out the periods of mania but it doesn't control the episodes of depression. If this is your problem, your doctor may combine Prozac (or another SSRI) with lithium. On the other hand, you shouldn't take Prozac without lithium if you have bipolar I manic-depression, since Prozac could push you into an out-of-control manic high. (Bipolar I is a severe form of manic-depression characterized by dark periods of deep depression alternating with highs so manic a person may require hospitalization.)

Who Shouldn't Take Lithium

You shouldn't take lithium if you have uncontrolled diabetes or untreated hypoglycemia (low blood sugar), or if you can't have your blood levels regularly tested. Nursing mothers and those allergic to lithium shouldn't take this medication either.

Who Benefits from Lithium

While the standard patient who takes lithium is diagnosed as a manic-depressive, it may also be given in combination with other antidepressants to a depressed person with a familial history of manic depression.

"My doctor wanted me to go on lithium because my brother is manic-depressive," says Eleanor, 38. "I didn't want to take it, because my brother takes lithium and he's really sick. I had an aversion to being diagnosed manic-depressive."

In fact, lithium alone did *not* help Eleanor, but when her psychiatrist combined it with the SSRI Paxil, her depression began to respond. "My psychiatrist says that Paxil helped my depression, and the lithium helped keep me from getting manic," she says. "I take 450 milligrams of lithium twice a day, and Paxil in the afternoon. I feel lighter. People started saying I look younger."

How to Take Lithium

Lithium will only work when it reaches the correct level in the bloodstream. The effective level of lithium is about the same for everybody. However, you can't just pop a pill and assume the lithium level is correct. Regular blood tests are necessary to make sure that the correct level of the drug is maintained. These tests are not only critical in determining whether the patient is getting enough lithium, but they also guard against getting too much. This is important because the level needed to correct mania and depression is very close to a level that can make you sick (see box: "Lithium Toxicity Symptoms").

Before you're given lithium, your doctor will probably arrange for some blood tests. You will probably receive annual monitoring that includes an EKG and a complete blood count. To guard against lithium toxicity, your doctor will need to measure the level of lithium in your blood to make sure you're not getting too much. This may seem inconvenient, but remember that inadequate monitoring can have fatal results. In the beginning, your doctor will probably monitor your blood level once a week until your dosage is stabilized, drawing blood levels 10–12 hours after your last dose. Once you're stabilized and taking maintenance therapy, your blood levels should be checked in a month, and then every three months.

To lessen the chance of stomach irritation, it's a good idea to take lithium with or after meals. It usually takes from one to three weeks to notice an improvement in your mania and several months to ease the depression. Patients experiencing acute mania are usually started out with at least 900 milligrams of lithium carbonate per day, although dosage is regulated according to blood levels and response.

Side Effects

More common and less dangerous side effects may include thirst and frequent urination. Some people also gain weight during the first few months they take lithium. A sensitivity to lithium might make you drowsy.

You should contact your doctor at the *first* sign of toxicity: drowsiness, sluggishness, unsteadiness, tremor, muscle twitching, vomiting or diarrhea. If you have a mild case of toxicity, your doctor will probably just discontinue lithium temporarily, and give you fluids and electrolytes. Because more severe cases can cause lasting brain damage or death, serious lithium poisoning usually requires aggressive treatment with hemodialysis.

If you have psoriasis or diabetes, you may notice your disease worsens during treatment with lithium.

Because it's important not to lose too much salt while you take lithium, be careful not to sweat too much, which can deplete body stores of salt and water and cause lithium toxicity. Avoid extremely hot climates and sauna baths for the same reason, and be careful of any illness that causes fever, sweating, vomiting, or diarrhea. This can also significantly alter the blood-lithium concentration, so you'll need to monitor blood levels if you get sick.

SIDE EFFECTS OF LITHIUM

COMMON

Anorexia	Shakiness
Diarrhea	Thirst
Dizziness	Tremor
Mouth dryness	Urination increase
Sexual problems	Vomiting

INFREQUENT

Acne	Weight gain
Ear noises	Shortness of breath
Fainting	Speech slurring
Fatigue	Stomach pain
Muscle aches	Heartbeat irregularities
Headache	Menstrual problems
Swelling	Rash (hands and feet)

Thyroid problems (coldness; dry, puffy skin)

RARE

Hair loss	Psoriasis worsening
Eye pain	Blurry vision
Arm and/or leg jerks	

If you're over age 60, you may have more frequent or severe side effects than younger people. Lithium isn't usually given to anyone under age 12.

Drug Interactions

It appears that while some people are good candidates for a lithium-Prozac combination, others aren't. While several reports have found that Prozac can interfere with lithium, the two drugs used together can help some depressed people who don't respond to either drug alone.

When taking lithium, you shouldn't take over-the-counter medications that contain iodide (such as some cough medicines and vitamin-mineral supplements), because these drugs may affect the thyroid when taken with lithium.

Use caution if you combine lithium with Tegretol, chlorpromazine (Thorazine), phenothiazines, Prozac, Haldol or methyldopa (Aldomet). In addition, lithium may increase the effects of tricyclic antidepressants.

The effects of lithium may be increased if you take Bumex, Edecrin, Prozac, furosemide (Lasix), Indocin, Feldene, or some diuretics. Some other drugs may decrease the effects of lithium, including acetazolamide (Diamox), sodium bicarbonate, theophylline (Theo-Dur).

There may be an increased risk of seizures by combining lithium with bupropion (Wellbutrin). Some drugs can also interact with lithium to produce toxicity, including some nonsteroidal anti-inflammatory drugs (such as ibuprofen).

Using cocaine or marijuana while taking lithium could cause psychosis.

Children and the Elderly

A safe effective level of lithium, as with many other antidepressants, hasn't been established for children under 12. If you're over age 60, you may need to take smaller-than-standard doses, beginning with a test dose of 75 to 150 milligrams daily. Be especially careful when taking lithium if you're on a low-salt diet and you use diuretics.

Pregnancy and Breast-feeding

Lithium therapy throughout the first trimester of pregnancy and beyond may be associated with birth defects (especially the heart). Studies have also shown that if the baby's blood level of lithium reaches toxic levels before birth, the child may have "floppy infant" syndrome (weakness, lethargy, unresponsiveness, low temperature, a weak cry, and poor appetite). Rat and mice pups exposed to lithium before birth have been born with defects of the ear, eye, and palate. *You should stop taking lithium immediately if you're trying to get pregnant, or if you've just conceived.*

Because lithium is found in breast milk in significant amounts, doctors also recommend that you not plan to nurse if you use lithium.

Dietary Restrictions

While you're taking lithium, you should never restrict your use of salt; too little could increase lithium's effect. Don't drink too much tea and coffee, which increases the risk of adverse effects. Drink plenty of liquids (at least 8 to 12 glasses of water each day), and don't skip meals. Don't drink alcohol at all with lithium.

Withdrawal

Suddenly stopping lithium medication doesn't cause any withdrawal symptoms. However, it's not a good idea to stop taking lithium too soon, since this may cause a return of either mania or depression. Some people may need treatment for at least a year. Don't stop taking lithium without talking to your doctor.

Long-Term Effects

Some people on long-term maintenance may experience altered thyroid function or goiter. Patients with kidney problems before starting on lithium often run into further kidney problems after using lithium for some time. (If you have kidney problems, you could either switch to Tegretol or Depakote.)

For some people with major depressive disorder and no history of mania or hypomania, Depakote alone can be very helpful in easing symptoms. In one recent study of three outpatients at the Dallas VA Mental Health Clinic, two-thirds of depressed patients responded well to the drug.

Your doctor may ask for follow-up medical exams or lab studies, such as an electrocardiogram, thyroid- or kidney-function tests, or complete blood counts.

Conclusion

We've seen how lithium can be of great help in the treatment of manic depression, especially early in the course of the disease. However, some experts believe that manic depression is a progressive disease that may worsen to the point where lithium just doesn't work anymore.

Even the alternative treatments (Tegretol and Depakote) may not fully control the symptoms of the disease in every person. For people like Jack, who was introduced at the beginning of this chapter, hope lies in the future, in some new drug that scientists may even now be testing. We'll discuss the latest information on new antidepressants in the pharmaceutical pipeline in the next chapter.

9
IN THE FUTURE

> *"I'm lithium-resistant and I don't respond very well to Tegretol or Depakote, so my only hope is for some new drug to be developed to treat manic depression. I don't care about side effects or what the drug might do 10 years from now. I need help now."*
>
> —Gerry, 53

The treatment of depression has come a long way in the past 40 years, but there are still problems to be overcome. Still needed are antidepressants with even fewer side effects and medications that will help the small percentage of depressed people who don't respond to any drug.

People like Gerry are counting on drug companies to come up with another "miracle drug"—like Prozac and the SSRIs—that will address his manic depression. He has good reason to be hopeful.

Analysts predict that by the end of the century, the market for antidepressants will double to more than $6 billion. Pharmaceutical manufacturers are poised on the brink of a virtual flood of new antidepressants ready to join today's $3-billion antidepressant market. According to the Pharmaceutical Research and Manufacturers of America, 16 medicines are currently being tested for mood disorders. But that doesn't mean that they'll all be on the market in the near future.

How a Drug is Born

On average, it takes 12 years for an experimental drug to travel from the laboratory to your medicine chest. Only 5 out of every 5,000 compounds that are initially tested make it to human testing; only one of these five is ever approved for human use.

The U.S. system of drug approvals is among the most stringent in the world, and it usually costs a company about $359 million to shepherd one medicine from the laboratory to the pharmacy, according to a 1993 report by the Congressional Office of Technology Assessment. The first step in the journey from drug lab to pharmacy shelf is preclinical testing, in which a drug company conducts animal and lab safety studies and determines how the compound works against a particular disease. These tests take about three-and-a-half years.

After completing this phase, a company files an "investigational new drug application" with the FDA for permission to test the drug on humans. The application shows the results of the preclinical testing and describes details about the upcoming studies, how the compound works, and any possible toxic effects. Once the application is approved, progress reports on clinical trials must be submitted yearly.

Next comes the year-long Phase I of the clinical trials in which 20 to 80 healthy volunteers test the drug for safety and to provide evidence of how the drug is absorbed, distributed, and excreted. Then comes about two years of Phase II effectiveness research involving between 100 and 300 volunteer patients who have the targeted disease. Phase III involves another three years of further tests of usefulness and side effects, and usually involves between 1,000 and 3,000 patients in clinics and hospitals.

Once all three phases of the clinical trials are over and the drug is considered to be safe and effective, the company files a New Drug Application (NDA), a document of more than 100,000 pages packed with all of the scientific data the company has gathered. Although by law the FDA must review the NDA within six months, the average review for approved compounds in 1993 took 26.5 months.

Once the FDA approves a new drug's application, the new medicine becomes available for doctors to prescribe. However, the drug company's job isn't over. It must still submit periodic reports to the FDA, including any information about side effects as they become known. For some drugs, the FDA requires more studies (called Phase IV) to evaluate long-term effects.

Once a drug is approved to treat a disease, physicians don't always prescribe it only for its approved use. For example, Prozac was initially approved just for the treatment of depression, but today physicians prescribe it for disorders ranging from migraines to shyness.

HOW TO JOIN A CLINICAL
ANTIDEPRESSANT TRIAL

If you've not found relief with any antidepressant, including tricyclics, MAOIs, and SSRIs, you have one final recourse: participating in a new antidepressant trial. Participation is free, and you'll receive close attention from highly qualified doctors during the trial.

➤ First step: Locate upcoming drug trial in radio, TV, or print ads.

➤ Telephone investigator for brief phone screening interview.

➤ If you're acceptable, you'll participate in a detailed psychiatric interview followed by a medical exam (including EKG).

➤ If eligible, you'll be asked to sign a two-page informed consent document.

➤ Phase I studies: Inpatients are treated with drugs in their earliest stage of development to determine dosages and safety.

➤ Phase II studies: Both in- and outpatients are given differing doses to check efficacy, tolerance, and side effects.

➤ Phase III studies: The new drug is compared to a placebo and one or two standard drugs.

➤ Phase IV: Drug studies take place after marketing to investigate the drug's usefulness with other diseases.

Upcoming Antidepressants

The next antidepressant you'll be hearing about is Luvox (fluvoxamine) for separate approval in each of the treatments of binge eating disorder, major depression and panic disorder.

Luvox has been approved by the FDA for use in treating obsessive-compulsive disorder. Already on sale in 36 countries, it is said to be as effective as Prozac in easing depression.

A host of other new compounds are in various stages of research. Currently in Phase III of the drug development process is flesinoxan, developed by Solvay Pharmaceuticals.

Drugs currently in Phase II of the antidepressant drug development process are

➤ amesergide and diluoxetine, both developed by Eli Lilly

➤ ipsapirone, developed by Miles, Inc.

➤ MDL 26, 479 developed by Marion Merrell Dow

➤ ORG 4428, developed by Organon

➤ roxindole (EMD 62100), developed by EM Industries.

Drugs currently in Phase I of the drug development process are

➤ BMS-181101, developed by Bristol-Myers Squibb

➤ SR-46349, SR-57227, and SR-58611, all developed by Elf Sanofi.

OTHER DISORDERS AND PROZAC

Prozac has been successfully used to ease a wide variety of symptoms and conditions, including:

Agoraphobia
Alcoholism
Anorexia nervosa
Body dysmorphic
  disorder
Borderline personality
  disorder
Bulimia
Dementia

Exhibitionism
Itchy skin
Nicotine withdrawal
Obsessive-complusive
  disorder
Panic Attacks
Premenstrual syndrome
Schizophrenia
Tourette's syndrome

At least 10 other antidepressants are under development and in use around the world, including Milnacipran, another serotonin-enhancer that resembles Effexor, and mianserin, a tetracyclic that acts on the serotonin and histamine systems. Tianeptine, a new tricyclic antidepressant without the side effects of classical tricyclics, was found to be helpful in treating depression according to a recent Brazilian study. Other new drugs include citalopram (an SSRI), brofaromine, Aurorix (moclobemide), Humeril (toloxotone), rolipram, dexfenfluramine and ritanserin. Some of these are already sold in Europe, and all are currently being studied in the United States.

In addition, some manufacturers of antidepressants already approved for the treatment of depression are now applying for approval to treat other disorders with the same drug.

Other Advances

Scientists are also studying ways not just to treat depression but to prevent its occurrence in vulnerable patients. They are currently searching for biological "markers"—a specific genetic code or psychological trait that may indicate who will become depressed. If people who carry this marker can be identified *before* their depression develops, they may be able to learn coping strategies to head off the disorder.

Herbal Preparations

The past few years have shown an increasing interest in herbal products to help with a variety of conditions including depression. The herbal extract *Hypericum perforatum*, commonly known as St. John's wort, has recently received considerable attention in the media. Many patients have begun to ask their psychiatrists if this herb could be a useful alternative to traditional antidepressant medication.

In Germany, St. John's wort is approved and widely used to treat depression, anxiety and sleep problems. But, since this herb is not FDA-approved in the United States and because most physicians have little or no experience prescribing it, most physicians are reluctant to recommend it.

The extract, which can be taken as a tea, liquid supplement, or capsule, is readily available in health food stores. The dosage range is between 250 to 900 mg per day.

It's not clear just how St. John's wort works. Side effects appear to be rare, but sensitivity to sunlight has been reported. As with other antidepressants, it may take between four to six weeks to work.

The August 1996 *British Medical Journal* presented an overview of the available data about St. John's wort and found that it is more effective than placebo for treating depression, although it isn't certain that the herb is as effective as other antidepressants. The article concluded that more research is needed.

Some other herbal preparations that are widely available but even less well researched include Kava Kava root *(Piper methysticum)*, passionflower *(Passiflora incarnata)*, Chinese schizandra berry *(Schizandra chinensis)*, wild oats *(Avena sativa)*, valerian root *(Valeriana officinalis)*, and the amino acid DLPA *(DL-phenylalanine)*.

Conclusion

The only thing more tragic than the thousands of depressed women and men in this country is the fact that so many of them are not being treated for their disorder. Far too many Americans still fear the stigma of the label of "mental illness." Others still believe that all antidepressants will make them dopey or groggy. Still others are just too depressed to find the energy to seek help.

The majority of mental health experts interviewed for this book agree that the new generation of antidepressants—not just Prozac, but Paxil, Zoloft, Wellbutrin and Effexor as well—is the best news yet for depressed patients. Given the new drugs' low toxicity and limited side effects, there's just no reason for any depressed person not to be given a chance at living a normal, healthy life.

GLOSSARY

adrenergic   Referring to the activation of neurons by catecholamine transmitters (such as epinephrine, norepinephrine, and dopamine).

agitated depression   A major depressive disorder characterized by restlessness, insomnia, and loss of appetite.

alprazolam   The generic name for Xanax, this is a benzodiazepine tranquilizer that may be useful for short-term treatment of minor depression.

amantadine   The generic name of Symmetrel.

amine   Organic compounds containing the amino group ($-NH_2$).

amino acids   Any organic acid containing one or more amino ($-NH_2$) groups; a basic part of proteins and the basic building blocks of neurotransmitters.

Anafranil   The brand name for clomipramine, this is a tricyclic antidepressant (also prescribed for obsessive-compulsive disorder).

anhedonia   Inability to experience pleasure from activities that usually produce pleasurable feelings.

antagonist   A drug that reduces or blocks the action of another drug.

antidepressant   A medication used to treat depression.

anticholinergic effects   The interference with the action of acetylcholine in the brain and peripheral nervous system by any drug. This term is often used to refer to the side effects of tricyclic antidepressants, such as dry mouth, blurred vision, and constipation.

anxiety   A feeling of apprehension, worry, or distress (often about events in the future); there may also be breathing problems, racing heartbeat, trembling, and sweating.

Artane   The brand name of trihexyphenidyl, a muscle relaxant used to treat Parkinsonism.

Asendin   The brand name of amoxapine, a tricyclic antidepressant.

Ativan   The brand name of lorazepam, an antianxiety medication also prescribed for anxiety with depression.

atypical bipolar II depression   A clinical condition in which periods of major depression alternate with periods of mild elation.

atypical depression   A type of depression in which the person reacts to the environment, is sensitive to rejection, and may gain weight and sleep more than usual; this condition is the opposite of typical depression, which is characterized by weight loss and insomnia.

Aventyl   The brand name of nortriptyline, a tricyclic antidepressant.

barbiturate   A habit-forming drug used to induce sleep or treat anxiety.

behavior therapy   A form of psychotherapy that seeks to modify behavior by manipulating the environment and behavior.

Benadryl   A nonprescription antihistamine used to treat allergies; it is also used to treat Parkinsonism.

benzodiazepines   A class of psychotropic drugs that have a hypnotic and sedative action, used mainly as tranquilizers for the control of symptoms due to anxiety or stress and as a sleeping aid for insomnia.

binge eating disorder   Episodic uncontrolled eating of large amounts of food without the purging that characterizes bulimia (binge-purge eating disorder).

biogenic amine hypothesis   The concept that abnormalities in the biogenic amines (especially the neurotransmitters norepinephrine, dopamine, and serotonin) are involved in depression. The idea was developed when researchers noticed that monoamine oxidase inhibitors and some tricyclic drugs were able to improve mood by affecting certain brain monoamine functions.

biogenic amines   Organic substances subdivided into catecholamines (epinephrine, dopamine, and norepinephrine) and indoles (tryptophan and serotonin), all of which appear to play a role in the development of depression.

bipolar disorder   A major affective disorder characterized by both mania and depression. A mild form of this disorder is sometimes called "cyclothymia." Bipolar disorders may be divided into manic, depressed, or mixed types on the basis of the patient's symptoms.

Manic type Symptoms are characterized by excitement, euphoria, expansive or irritable mood, hyperactivity, pressured speech, flight of ideas, limited sleep needs, distractibility, impaired judgment. There may be grandiose or elated delusions.

Depressed type Symptoms are characterized by slow thinking, lowered mood, decreased movement or agitation, loss of interest, guilt, negative self-esteem, sleep problems, appetite loss.

Mixed type Symptoms of mania and depression occur at the same time.

bipolar I disorder Also known as manic depression, this is a clinical condition characterized by alternating episodes of major depression and mania or elation often severe enough to require hospitalization.

bipolar II disorder A clinical condition characterized by alternating periods of major depression and mild mania. A patient may need to be hospitalized during depressed periods but usually not during the manic phase.

bipolar III A term used to describe a depressed person who develops mild or severe mania only after taking certain drugs (such as antidepressants).

bupropion The generic name for Wellbutrin, an antidepressant drug.

BuSpar The brand name of buspirone, this is a nonhabit-forming antianxiety medication.

buspirone The generic name for BuSpar, a nonhabit-forming antianxiety medication.

carbamazepine The generic name for Tegretol.

chloral hydrate The generic name for Noctec, a sleeping medication.

cholinergic Activated by acetylcholine.

citalopram The name for an SSRI antidepressant currently being developed.

clinical depression A medical term often used for major depression.

clomipramine The generic name for Anafranil, a tricyclic antidepressant.

clonidine An antihypertensive (high blood pressure) drug also used for narcotic withdrawal.

chlorpromazine The generic name for Thorazine.

Cogentin The brand name for benztropine, a medication used to treat Parkinsonism.

cognitive therapy A structured form of short-term psychotherapy in which the goal is to change the negative, inaccurate ways of thinking.

Coumadin The brand name for warfarin, a blood-thinning medication.

cyclothymia A form of manic depression characterized by relatively mild highs and lows.

Cytomel A thyroid hormone sometimes used to boost the effectiveness of an antidepressant.

Dalmane   The brand name of flurazepam, a benzodiazepine drug used as a hypnotic agent or sleeping pill.

Depakote   The brand name for valproic acid, this is an anticonvulsant drug and an alternative to lithium for the treatment of manic depression.

Deprenyl   A European monoamine oxidase inhibitor that lacks the "cheese effect" (harmful interaction with cheese and other tyramine-containing food), which is used to treat Parkinson's disease.

depressive illness   Endogenous depression characterized by depressed mood (sadness, hopelessness, etc.), reduced energy level (fatigue, loss of interest, etc.), and negative self-image. Common features include sleep problems, early awakening, loss of appetite, etc.

depressive reaction   A reactive depression that represents an understandable response to a significant loss or stressful life situation, involving a sense of despondency and distress. It is usually comparatively mild to moderate and usually passes within two weeks to six months.

desipramine   The generic name for Norpramin, a tricyclic antidepressant.

Desyrel   The brand name for trazodone, an antidepressant structurally unlike the tricyclics, MAOIs, and SSRIs.

diazepam   The generic name for Valium.

dopamine   One of the major neurotransmitters found in the synapses of the brain; low levels of dopamine are associated with depression.

double depression An episode of major depression that occurs in addition to a chronic, long-term mild depression.

DSM-IV An abbreviation for the fourth edition of the *Diagnostic and Statistical Manual of Mental Disorders* published by the *American Psychiatric Association. DSM-IV* lists all symptoms for all psychiatric disorders.

dysphoria An unpleasant mood associated with a shifting set of symptoms including sadness, anxiety, and irritability.

dysthymic disorder This mild but persistent form of depression is also called "depressive neurosis," a chronic disturbance of mood involving depression *for at least two years* (one year in children). In addition, symptoms include poor appetite or overeating, insomnia or excessive fatigue, low energy, poor self-esteem, poor concentration, hopelessness.

Effexor The brand name for venlafaxine, an antidepressant.

elation A strong feeling of exhilaration, euphoria, and optimism.

Elavil The brand name for amitriptyline, a tricyclic antidepressant.

endogenous depression A spontaneous, unexplained, and seemingly unprovoked depression of moderate to severe degree.

epinephrine Also known as adrenaline, this is one of the catecholamines secreted by the adrenal gland and the sympathetic nervous system responsible for physical symptoms of fear and anxiety.

fluoxetine The generic name for Prozac, an SSRI antidepressant.

fluvoxamine The generic name for Luvox, an SSRI antidepressant.

generic drugs A drug not controlled by a manufacturer's trademark.

Halcion The brand name for triazolam, a short-acting benzodiazepine hypnotic or sleeping pill.

Haldol The brand name for haloperidol, an antipsychotic drug.

hyperthymia A mood characterized by high energy, confidence, and activity; it is more energetic than a normal mood but less so than mild forms of mania (hypomania).

hypomania A mildly elevated mood lasting a few days, less intense than mania but more intense than hyperthymia.

hypothalamus A part of the brain responsible for regulating automatic activities of the body, such as hunger, thirst, body temperature, and sexual activity.

imipramine The generic name for Tofranil, a tricyclic antidepressant.

interpersonal psychotherapy A type of structured short-term therapy designed to treat depression.

isocarboxazid The generic name for Marplan, an antidepressant MAO inhibitor.

L-tryptophan An amino acid used to make serotonin.

levodopa   The precursor of dopamine; as a drug, this is used to treat Parkinson's disease.

Librium   The brand name for chlordiazepoxide, an antianxiety drug and member of the benzodiazepine family.

lithium   An element which, when used as a medication, can stabilize fluctuating ups and downs of mood disorders by shifting the levels of water and electrolytes.

Ludiomil   The brand name for maprotiline, a tetracyclic antidepressant.

Luvox   The brand name for fluvoxamine, an SSRI antidepressant.

major affective disorder   A group of disorders with a persistent, prominent disturbance of mood (depression or mania) and a full syndrome of symptoms; major depression and bipolar disorder are both examples of major affective disorder.

major depressive episode   Also known as clinical or unipolar depression, or major depressive disorder, this is an episode lasting at least two weeks, characterized by at least four of the following symptoms: loss of ability to experience pleasure and interest, fatigue, feelings of worthlessness or guilt, concentration problems, appetite and sleep disturbances, frequent thoughts of suicide and death. If at least four of these symptoms are present *in addition* to at least one episode of mania, then the diagnosis becomes bipolar disorder (or manic-depressive illness).

mania   A period of persistent elation characterized by hyperactivity, agitation, rapid talking, excitement, or flight of ideas.

manic-depressive illness   A disorder characterized by alternating episodes of moderate to severe depression and unstable periods of elation. It is also known as bipolar I disorder. The periods of mania are distinct, with a predominant mood that is elevated, expansive, or irritable. Other symptoms of mania include hyperactivity, flight of ideas, inflated self-esteem, little need for sleep, distractibility, and excessive involvement in activities that may be flamboyant, bizarre, or disorganized.

MAOI   The abbreviation for monoamine oxidase inhibitor, a type of antidepressant.

maprotiline   The generic name for Ludiomil, a tetracyclic antidepressant.

Marplan   The brand name for isocarboxazid, an MAO inhibitor.

masked depression   A type of depression hidden behind physical symptoms with no apparent physical cause.

melancholia   A term used to refer to a severe form of depression. In psychiatric diagnoses, "major depression with melancholia" refers to a severe depression including loss of pleasure, worse morning moods, psychomotor retardation or agitation, weight loss, and insomnia.

Mellaril   The brand name for thioridazine, an antipsychotic drug used rarely for the short-term treatment of depression with anxiety.

metabolite   The chemical compound produced by the breakdown of a drug in the body.

methylphenidate (Ritalin)   Drug often used to treat hyperactive children that may be tried for long-term treatment of selected elderly people with depression.

MHPG (3-methoxy-4-hydroxyphenylglycol)   A major metabolite of norepinephrine excreted in urine; low MHPG levels occur in depression, while high levels are found in bipolar patients during manic phases. Research suggests that MHPG levels may be used to classify depression types and to predict responses to tricyclic antidepressants.

Mianserin   A tetracyclic antidepressant available in Europe but not yet approved in the United States.

mirtazapine   The generic name for the antidepressant Remeron.

monoamine oxidase (MAO)   An enzyme that breaks down biogenic amines (neurotransmitters). Inhibition of this enzyme by certain antidepressant drugs (MAO inhibitors) may relieve a patient's depression.

monoamine oxidase inhibitor (MAOI)   A class of antidepressants that keeps the enzyme monoamine oxidase from breaking down, resulting in higher levels of norepinephrine and serotonin at the nerve synapses.

mood (affective) disorders   A group of clinical conditions characterized by feelings of lack of control over mood or emotions, primarily depression and mania. Mood disorders can affect basic functions such as cognitive ability, sleep patterns, appetite, and sexuality, and can interfere with personal and professional life.

mood episode A mood syndrome that has no known organic cause and that is not part of a psychotic disorder (such as schizophrenia). A mood episode can be either major depressive, manic, or hypomanic.

mood syndrome A group of mood and associated symptoms that occur together for a minimum amount of time. Mood syndromes can occur as part of a mood disorder, a psychotic disorder, or an organic mental disorder.

Nardil The brand name for phenelzine, an MAOI antidepressant.

nefazadone The generic name for the antidepressant Serzone.

neuron A nerve cell.

neurotransmitter A chemical in the nervous system (such as dopamine or serotonin) that carries messages across the gaps (synapses) between neurons. Dysfunction in this neurotransmitter system has been linked to depression.

norepinephrine Also called noradrenaline, this is one of the three major neurotransmitters found in the brain and implicated in the development of depression. High levels of this substance in the brain have been linked to manic states; low levels have been linked to depression.

norfluoxetine A metabolite of Prozac.

normal reactive depression   A short-term depression caused by grief or bereavement.

Norpramin   The brand name for desipramine, a tricyclic antidepressant.

nortriptyline   The generic name for the tricyclic anti-depressants Pamelor and Aventyl.

obsessive-compulsive disorder   A clinical condition characterized by distressing repetition of thoughts that are intense, frightening, absurd, or unusual, together with ritualized actions that are usually bizarre and irrational.

orthostatic hypotension   A precipitous fall in blood pressure upon sitting or standing up, causing dizziness or fainting. This is a common side effect in some antidepressants.

Pamelor   The brand name for nortriptyline, a tricyclic antidepressant.

Parnate   The brand name for tranylcypromine, an MAOI antidepressant.

paroxetine   The generic name for Paxil, an SSRI antidepressant.

Paxil   The brand name for paroxetine, an SSRI antidepressant.

phenelzine   The generic name for Nardil, an MAOI antidepressant.

phenothiazine   A generic name for a family of antipsychotic drugs including Thorazine, Stelazine, and Mellaril.

protriptyline The generic name for Vivactil, a tricyclic antidepressant.

Prozac The trade name for fluoxetine, an SSRI antidepressant.

psychotropic drugs Medications that affect mood or mental activity.

rapid cyclers Manic-depressive people who experience more than four mood swings a year.

Remeron The brand name for mirtazipine, a new antidepressant that works on norepinephrine and serotonin.

selective serotonin reuptake inhibitors (SSRIs) A class of antidepressants that work by blocking the reabsorption of serotonin in the brain, raising the levels of serotonin. SSRIs include Prozac, Zoloft, and Paxil.

Serzone The brand name for nefazadone, a serotonin-related antidepressant that is similar to an SSRI..

serotonin One of the three major neurotransmitters found in the synapses of the brain linked to the development of depression.

sertraline The generic name for Zoloft, an SSRI antidepressant.

soft bipolar A form of mania or hypomania that is too mild to meet the requirements of a formal *DSM-IV* diagnosis.

SSRI Selective serotonin reuptake inhibitor.

Stelazine   The brand name for trifluoperazine, a major antipsychotic or tranquilizer of the phenothiazine family.

subclinical depression   A form of depression not severe enough to meet the diagnostic criteria for major depression or dysthymia.

Surmontil   The brand name for trimipramine, a tricyclic antidepressant.

Survector   The brand name for amineptine, an antidepressant available in Europe.

synapse   The gap between two nerve cells at which the transmission of nerve impulses occurs.

Tegretol   The brand name for carbamazepine, an anticonvulsant drug and an alternative to lithium for the treatment of manic-depression.

tetracyclic antidepressant   A class of antidepressants named for their four-ring chemical structure. Ludiomil is an example of a tetracyclic.

Tofranil   The brand name for imipramine, the first tricyclic antidepressant.

tranylcypromine   The generic name for Parnate, an MAOI antidepressant.

trazodone   The generic name for Desyrel, an antidepressant.

treatment-resistant depression   Depression that is not affected by any of the major classes of antidepressants.

tricyclic antidepressant   A class of antidepressants named for their three-ring chemical structure. TCAs increase the level of norepinephrine and serotonin in the synapses of the brain.

unipolar psychoses   Recurrent major depressions.

Valium   The brand name of diazepam, this is an antianxiety medication and minor tranquilizer.

valproic acid   The generic name for Depakote, an anticonvulsive medication used to treat manic depression.

venlafaxine   The generic name for Effexor, a new SSRI antidepressant.

vesicle   A small saclike structure that forms the brain during fetal development.

Vivactil   The brand name for protriptyline, a tricyclic antidepressant.

Wellbutrin   The brand name for bupropion, an antidepressant with a structure unlike SSRIs, MAOIs, or tricyclics.

withdrawal   The process of stopping a drug.

Xanax   The brand name for alprazolam, an antianxiety medication and minor tranquilizer.

Zoloft   The brand name for sertraline, an SSRI antidepressant.

REFERENCES

"ABCs of Antidepressants," *USA Today* 121(February 1993): 12.

Ablow, Russell Keith. "Prozac: What Kind of Cure?" *Washington Post* 115(February 11, 1992): WH9.

"Advances in the Diagnosis and Management of Depres-sion: Part I," *American Pharmacy* NS28(1): January 1988.

Ahmad, S. R. "USA: Fluoxetine 'Not Linked to Suicide,'" *The Lancet* 338(October 5, 1951): 875–6.

Akiskal, H.S., et al. "The Nosological Status of Neurotic Depression." Archives of General Psychiatry 35(1978): 756–66.

———, "The prevalent clinical spectrum of bipolar disorders: beyond DSM-IV," *Journal of Clinical Psychopharmacology* 16(April 1996): 4S–14S.

———, et al. "Psychopathology, Temperament and Past Course in Primary Major Depressions," *Psychopathology* 22(5)(1989): 268–77.

———, Downs, John, et al. "Affective Disorders in Referred Children and Younger Siblings of Manic Depressives: Mode of Onset and Prospective Course," *Archives of General Psychiatry* 42(1985): 996–1003.

———, and R. Haykal. "Fluoxetine Found Effective for Dysthymia," *Clinical Psychiatry News* 20/2(February 1992): 4F.

———, "New Insight into the Nature and Heterogeneity of Mood Disorders," *Journal of Clinical Psychiatry* 50(supp)(May 1990): 6–10, 11–2.

————. "The Clinical Spectrum of So-Called 'Minor' Depressions," *American Journal of Psychotherapy.* 46(1)(1992): 9–22.

American Psychiatric Association: *Diagnostic and Statistical Manual of Mental Disorders IV-R.* Washington, D.C., 1994.

American Psychological Association. *Factsheet: Women and Depression.* Washington, D.C.

Angier, Natalie. "Can a Pill Called Prozac End Depression?" *Mademoiselle,* April 1990, 229–32.

Austin, Linda, et al. "Rapid Response of Patients Simultaneously Treated with Lithium and Nortriptyline," *Journal of Clinical Psychiatry* 51(1990): 124–5.

Baldessarini, Ross J. "Fluoxetine and Side Effects," *Archives of General Psychiatry* 47(1990): 191–2.

Balon, Richard, et al. "Sexual Dysfunction During Antidepressant Treatment," *Journal of Clinical Psychiatry* 54(June 1993): 67.

Barefoot, J.C., et al, "Depression and long-term mortality risk in patients with coronary artery disease," *American Journal of Cardiology* 78(September 15, 1996): 613–617.

Baxter, Lewis R., Jeffrey M. Schwartz, et al. "Caudate Glucose Metabolic Rate Changes with Both Drug and Behavior Therapy for Obsessive-Compulsive Disorder," *Archives of General Psychiatry* 49(1992): 681–89.

Beasley, C. M., B. E. Dornseif, et al. "Fluoxetine and Suicide: a Meta-analysis of Controlled Trials of Treatment for Depression," *British Medical Journal* 303(1991): 685–92.

Begley, Sharon. "One Pill Makes You Larger, and One Pill Makes You Small." *Newsweek,* February 7, 1994, 36–40.

Berrettinni, Wade, et al. "X-Chromosome Markers and Manic-Depressive Illness," *Archives of General Psychiatry* 47(April 1990): 366–73.

Bihm, B., and B.A. Wilson, "Understanding fluoxetine (Prozac)," *Medsurgical Nursing* 5(February 1996): 50–52, 56.

Bittman, B. J., and R. C. Young. "Mania in Elderly Man Treated with Bupropion," Letter, *American Journal of Psychiatry* 148(4)(1991): 541.

Bloomfield, Harold, and Peter McWilliams. *How to Heal Depression,* Los Angeles: Prelude Press, 1994.

Bodkin, J. A., and M. H. Teicher. "Fluoxetine May Antagonize the Anxiolytic Action of Buspirone," *Journal of Clinical Psychopharmacology* 9 (2)(April 1989): 150.

de Boer, T.H., et al, "Differences in modulation of noradrenergic and serotonergic transmission by the alpha-2 adrenoreceptor antagonists, mirtazapine, mianserin and idazoxan," *Journal of Pharmacological Experimental Therapy* 277(May 1996): 852–60.

Bohn, J., and J. W. Jefferson. *Lithium and Manic Depression: A Guide* (revised edition), Madison, WI: Lithium Information Center, 1990.

Borys, D. J., et al. "Acute Fluoxetine Overdose: A Report of 234 Cases," *Journal of Emergency Medicine* 10(2)(1992): 115–20.

Boulos, C., et al. "An Open Naturalistic Trial of Fluoxetine in Adolescents and Young Adults with Treatment-Resistant Major Depression," *Journal of Child and Adolescent Psychopharmacology* 2(2)(1992): 103–111.

Bowe, Claudia. "Women and depression: Are we being overdosed?" *Redbook*, March 1992, 42–5.

Bower, Bruce. "Drugs, Depression and Molecular Ferries," *Science News* 140(Oct. 26, 1991): 261.

Brandes, L. J., R. J. Arron, et al. "Stimulation of Malignant Growth in Rodents by Antidepressant Drugs at Clinically Relevant Doses," *Cancer Research* 52(1992): 3796–3800.

Brendler, John, Michael Silver, Madlynn Haber, and John Sargent. *Madness, Chaos and Violence: Therapy with Families at the Brink,* New York: Basic Books, 1991.

Brodaty, Henry, Karin Peters, et al. "Age and Depression," *Journal of Affective Disorders* 23(1991): 137–49.

Brown, C., et al, "Treatment outcomes for primary care patients with major depression and lifetime anxiety disorders," *American Journal of Psychiatry* 153(October 1996): 1293–1300.

Bunney, W .E., and J. Davis. "Norepinephrine in Depressive Reactions." *Archives of General Psychiatry* 13(1965): 483–94.

Burns, David. *Feeling Good: The New Mood Therapy,* New York: Signet, 1980.

Cabrera-Vera, T.M., et al, "Effect of prenatal fluoxetine (Prozac) exposure on brain serotonin neurons in prepubescent and adult male rat offspring," *Journal of Pharmacology Experimental Therapy* 280(January 1997): 138–45.

Cohen, Bennet J., et al. "More Cases of SIADH with Fluoxetine," *American Journal of Psychiatry* 147(7)(July 1990): 948–9.

"Committee Advises FDA on Antidepressants," *FDA Consumer* 25(December 1991): 5.

Costa e Silva, et al, "Placebo-controlled study of tianeptine in major depressive episodes," *Neuropsychobiology* 35(1997): 24–9.

Cowen, R. "Sociopaths, Suicide and Serotonin," *Science News* 136(October 14, 1989): 250.

———. "Receptor Encounters: Untangling the Threads of the Serotonin System," *Science News* 136(October 14, 1989): 248–50, 252.

Cowley, Geoffrey. "The Promise of Prozac," *Newsweek*, March 26, 1990, 38–41.

———. "A Prozac Backlash: Does America's Favorite Antidepressant Make Some People Crazy?" *Newsweek*, April 1, 1991, 64–7.

———. "The Culture of Prozac: How a Treatment for Depression Became as Familiar as Kleenex and as Socially Acceptable as Spring Water," *Newsweek*, Feb. 7, 1994, 41–2.

Cunningham, Malcolm, et al. "Eye Tics and Subjective Hearing Impairment During Fluoxetine Therapy," *American Journal of Psychiatry* 147(7)(July 1990): 947–8.

Damluji, N. F., and J. M. Ferguson. "Paradoxical Worsening of Depressive Symptomatology Caused by Antidepressants," *Journal of Clinical Psychopharmacology* 8(5)(1988): 347–9.

Danish University Antidepressant Group. "Paroxetine: A Selective Serotonin Reuptake Inhibitor Showing Better Tolerance, but Weaker Antidepressant Effect Than Clomipramine in a Controlled Multicenter Study," *Journal of Affective Disorders* 18(1990): 289–99.

Davis, Lori, et al, "Valproate as an antidepressant in major depressive disorder," *Psychopharmacology Bulletin* 32(4)(1996): 647–52.

Delgado, Pedro, et al. "Serotonin Function and the Mechanism of Antidepressant Action: Reversal of Antidepressant-Induced Remission by Rapid Depletion of Plasma Tryptophan," *Archives of General Psychiatry* 47(1990): 411–18.

Denniston, Philip, ed. *1993 Physicians' GenRX: Official Drug Reference of the FDA,* New York: Data Pharmaceutica, 1993.

"Depressing Danger," *Time*, May 17, 1993, 5.

Divish, Margaret, et al. "Differential Effect of Lithium on Fos Protooncogene Expression Mediated by Receptor and Postreceptor Activators of Protein Kinase C and Cyclic Adenosine Monophosphate: Model for Its Antimanic Action," *Journal of Neuroscience Research* 28 (1991): 40–48.

Dowling, Colette. *You Mean I Don't Have to Feel This Way?* New York: Charles Scribner's Sons, 1991.

Duke, Patty. *A Brilliant Madness: Living with Manic-Depressive Illness,* New York: Bantam Books, 1992.

Eichelman, Burr. "Aggressive Behavior: From Laboratory to Clinic: Quo vadit?" *Archives of General Psychiatry* 49/6(June 1992): 488–92.

Eisenberg, Leon. "Treating Depression and Anxiety in Primary Care: Closing the Gap Between Knowledge and Practice," *New England Journal of Medicine* 326(1992): 1080–84.

Elmer-Dewitt, Philip. "Depression: The Growing Role of Drug Therapies," *Time*, July 6, 1992, 56–9.

Emptage, R.E., and T.P. Semia, "Depression in the medically ill elderly; a focus on methylphenidate," *Annals of Pharmacotherapy* 30(February 1996): 151–7.

Extein, Irl, et al. *New Medicines of the Mind,* New York: Berkley Books, 1990.

Falk, William. "Suit: Drug Prompted Suicide Attempts," *Newsday,* July 18, 1990, 8.

Fava, Maurizio, and Jerold Rosenbaum. "Suicidality and Fluoxetine: Is There a Relationship?" *Journal of Clinical Psychiatry* 52(March 1991): 108–111.

———, "Does Fluoxetine Increase the Risk of Suicide?" *The Harvard Mental Health Letter* 7(7)(January 1991): 8.

———, et al. "Antidepressants Found to Prevent Depression-Related 'Anger Attacks,'" *Clinical Psychiatry News* (September 1992): 6.

Feder, R. "Fluoxetine-Induced Mania," *Journal of Clinical Psychiatry* 51(12)(1990): 524–5.

Feighner, J. P. "A Comparative Trial of Fluoxetine and Amitriptyline in Patients With Major Depressive Disorder," *Journal of Clinical Psychiatry* 46(1985): 369–372.

Fieve, Ronald. *Prozac: Questions and Answers for Patients, Family and Physicians,* New York: Avon Books, 1994.

———. *Moodswing,* New York: William Morrow, 1989.

Fink, Max. "Can ECT Be an Effective Treatment for Adolescents?" *Harvard Mental Health Letter* 10(11)(1994): 8.

———. *Convulsive Therapy: Theory and Practice,* New York: Raven Press, 1979.

Fleming, Jan, and David R. Offord, "Epidemiology of Childhood Depressive Disorders: A Critical Review," *Journal of the American Academy of Child and Adolescent Psychiatry* 29(4)(July 1990): 571–80.

Frank, Ellen, et al. "Three-Year Outcomes for Maintenance Therapies in Recurrent Depression," *Archives of General Psychiatry* 47(December 1990): 1093–99.

Frankel, K.A., and R.J. Harmon, "Depressed mothers: they don't always look as bad as they feel," *Journal of the American Academy of Child and Adolescent Psychiatry* 35(March 1996): 289–98.

Franklin, Deborah. "The Ups and Downs of Prozac," *In Health,* January/February 1991, 24–25.

Franklin, Erica. "Treating Anxiety Like the Blues," *American Health,* March 1990, 46.

Freeman, S. J., M. K. Oneil, and W. J. Lance. "Sex Differences in Depression in University Students," *Social Psychiatry* 20(4)(1985): 184–190.

Freeman, Hugh. "Meclobemide," *The Lancet* 342(December 18, 1993): 1528–32.

Gelman, David. "Drugs vs. the Couch," *Newsweek,* March 26, 1990, 42–43.

Glassman, Alexander, et al. "The Safety of Tricyclic Antidepressants in Cardiac Patients: Risk-Benefit Reconsidered," *JAMA* 269 (May 26, 1993): 2673–5.

Goff, D. C., A. W. Brotman, et al. " Trial of Fluoxetine Added to Neuroleptics for Treatment-Resistant Schizophrenic Patients," *American Journal of Psychiatry* 147(4)(April 1990): 492–4.

Gold, Mark. *The Good News About Depression,* New York: Bantam Books, 1986.

Goode, Erica. "Beating Depression," *US News & World Report* (March 5, 1990): 48–51, 53, 55–56.

Goodwin, Frederick, and Kay Redfield Jamison. *Manic-Depressive Illness,* New York: Oxford University Press, 1990.

Gorman, Jack. *The Essential Guide to Psychiatric Drugs*, New York: St. Martin's Press, 1990.

Grady, Denise. "Wonder Drug/Killer Drug: The Furor Over Prozac Won't Go Away," *American Health*, October 1990, 60–65.

Greist, John, and James Jefferson. *Depression and Its Treatment*, New York: Warner Books, 1992.

———. *Dealing with Depression: Taking Steps in the Right Direction*, New York: Pfizer, 1992.

Griffin, Katherine. "The Unbearable Darkness of Being," *In Health*, January/February 1991, 62–6.

Griffith, H. Winter. *Complete Guide to Prescription and Non-Prescription Drugs*, New York: The Putnam Publishing Group, 1992.

Hadley, A., and M. P. Cason. "Mania Resulting from Lithium-Fluoxetine Combination, Letter, *American Journal of Psychiatry* 146(1989): 1637–8.

Hamilton, J. A., B. L. Parry, and S. J. Blumenthal. "The Menstrual Cycle in Context I: Affective Syndromes Associated With Reproductive Hormonal Changes," *Journal of Clinical Psychiatry*, March 1988.

Hanna, M. E., et al. "Severe Lithium Toxicity Associated With Indapamide Therapy," *Journal of Clinical Psychopharmacology* 10(1990): 379.

Harkness, Richard. *Drug Interactions Guide Book*, Englewood Cliffs, NJ: Prentice Hall, 1991.

Harvey, K.V., and R.Balon, "Clinical implications of antidepressant drug effects on sexual function," *Annals of Clinical Psychiatry* 7(December 1995): 189–201.

Hellerstein, D. J., et al. "A Randomized Double-Blind Study of Fluoxetine Versus Placebo in the Treatment of Dysthymia," *American Journal of Psychiatry* 150(8)(1993): 1169–1975.

Herman, John B., et al. "Fluoxetine-Induced Sexual Dysfunction," *Journal of Clinical Psychiatry* 51(January 1990): 25–27.

"High Anxiety," *Consumer Reports* 58(January 1993): 19–24.

Higley, J. Dee, P. T. Mehlman, et al. "Cerebrospinal Fluid Monoamine and Adrenal Correlates of Aggression in Free-Ranging Rhesus Monkeys," *Archives of General Psychiatry* 49(6)(June 1992): 436–41.

Hirschfield, R.M.A., et al, "The National Depressive and Manic-Depressive Association consensus statement on the undertreatment of depression," *JAMA* 277(January 22–29, 1997): 333–40.

Holden, C. "Depression: The News Isn't Depressing," *Science* 254(1991): 1450–1452.

Hollander, Eric, and Allison McCarley. "Yohimbine Treatment of Sexual Side Effects Induced by Serotonin Reuptake Blockers," *Journal of Clinical Psychiatry* 53(1992): 207–9.

Hoover, C. E. "Suicidal Ideation Not Associated With Fluoxetine," Letter, *American Journal of Psychiatry* 148(1991): 543.

Jefferson, James, and John Greist. *Depression and Adolescents: Recognizing the Signs of Depression and Taking Steps to Help,* New York: Pfizer, April 1993.

———. *Depression and Older People: Recognizing Hidden Signs and Taking Steps Toward Recovery,* New York: Pfizer, 1993.

Jerome, L. "Hypomania with Fluoxetine," *Journal of American Academy of Child and Adolescent Psychiatry* 30(5)(1991): 850–1.

Joffe, et al. "Clinical Features of Situational and Nonsituational Major Depression," *Psychopathology* 26(3-4)(1993): 138–144.

Jonas, Jeffrey, and Ron Schaumburg. *Everything You Need to Know About Prozac*, New York: Bantam Books, 1991.

Kalasapudi, Vasundhara D., et al. "Lithium Augments Fos Protooncogene Expression in PC12 Pheochromocytoma Cells: Implications for Therapeutic Action of Lithium," *Brain Research* 521(1990): 47–54.

Kapur, Shitij, et al. "Antidepressant Medications and the Relative Risk of Suicide Attempt and Suicide," *JAMA* 268(December 23, 1992): 3441-5.

Karasu, T. Byrum. "Toward a Clinical Model of Psychotherapy for Depression II: An Integrative and Selective Treatment Approach," *American Journal of Psychiatry* 147(March 1990): 269-78.

Kendler, K. S., et al. "Major Depression and Generalized Anxiety Disorder: Same Genes, (Partly) Different Environments?" *Archives of General Psychiatry* 49(1992): 716–722.

Kendler, K. S. "Risk Factors in the Familial Aggregation of Psychiatric Disorders," *Psychosomatic Medicine* 20(2)(1990): 311–319.

Klein, D. F., and P. H. Wender. *Understanding Depression: A Complete Guide to Its Diagnosis and Treatment*, New York: Oxford University Press, 1993.

Klerman, G. L., and M. M. Weisman. "Increasing Rates of Depression," *JAMA* 261(1989): 2229–35.

Kline, Nathan. *From Sad to Glad: Kline on Depression*, New York: Putnam, 1974.

Koren, G., "First trimester exposure to fluoxetine (Prozac). Does it affect pregnancy outcome?" *Canadian Family Physician* 42(January 1996): 43–4.

Kovacs, Maria, Terry L. Feinberg, et al. "Depressive Disorders in Childhood," *Archives of General Psychiatry* 41(July 1984): 646.

Kramer, Peter. *Listening to Prozac,* New York: Viking Press, 1993.

Kupfer, David J. "Long-term Treatment of Depression," *Journal of Clinical Psychiatry* 52(5)(May 1991): 28–34.

Larkin, Ellen. "Depression and Advancing Age," *FDA Consumer* 27(March 1993): 18–22.

Leibenluft, E., "Women with bipolar illness: clinical and research issues," *American Journal of Psychiatry* 153(February 1996): 163–73

Liebowitz, M. R., E. Hollander, et al. "Fluoxetine for Adolescents with Obsessive-Compulsive Disorder," *American Journal of Psychiatry* 147(3)(March 1990): 370–1.

"Lifetime and Twelve-Month Prevalence of DSM-III-R Psychiatric Disorders in the United States," *Archives of General Psychiatry* 51(January 1994): 8–19.

Linde, Klaus, et al, "St. John's wort for depression—an overview and metaanalysis of randomised clinical trials," *British Medical Journal* 313(1996): 253–8.

Long, James. *Essential Guide to Prescription Drugs,* New York: HarperCollins, 1994.

Maj, Mario, Franco Veltro, et al. "Pattern of Recurrence of Illness After Recovery from an Episode of Major Depression: A Prospective Study," *American Journal of Psychiatry* 149(June 1992): 795–800.

Mann, J. J., Anne McBride, et al. "Relationship Between Central and Peripheral Serotonin Indexes in Depressed and Suicidal Psychiatric Inpatients" *Archives of General Psychiatry* 49/6(June 1992): 442–59.

Mann, J. J., and S. Kapur. "The Emergence of Suicidal Ideation and Behavior During Antidepressant Therapy," *Archives of General Psychiatry* 48(November 1991): 1027–33.

Marcus, M. D., R. R. Wing, et al. "A Double-Blind, Placebo-Controlled Trial of Fluoxetine Plus Behavior Modification in the Treatment of Obese Binge-Eaters and Non-Binge-Eaters," *American Journal of Psychiatry* 147(7)(July 1990): 876–81.

Markovitz, P. J., S. J. Stagno, and J. R. Calabrese. "Buspirone Augmentation of Fluoxetine in Obsessive-Compulsive Disorder," *American Journal of Psychiatry* 147(6)(June 1990): 798–800.

Marx, Jean. "Do Antidepressants Promote Tumors?" *Science* 257 (July 3, 1992): 22–23.

McCoy, Kathleen. *Coping with Teenage Depression,* New York: Penguin, 1982.

McEnay, Geoffrey. "Nursing the Mind: Managing Mood Disorders," *RN* 53(September 1990): 28–33.

McGrath, Ellen. *When Feeling Bad Is Good,* New York: Bantam Books, 1994.

McKnew, Donald, Leon Cytryn, and Herbert Yahraes. *Why Isn't Johnny Crying?* New York: W. W. Norton, 1983.

Milani, R.V., et al, "Effects of cardiac rehabilitation and exercise training programs on depression in patients after major coronary events," *American Heart Journal* 132(October 1996): 726–32.

Minear, Ralph. *Kids' Symptoms from Birth to Teens,* New York: Avon Books, 1992.

Mitka, Mike. "Drug Maker to Defend Physicians Sued over Prozac," *American Medical News* 34(June 24, 1991): 14.

Moore, Jeffrey, and Robert Rodriguez. "Toxicity of Fluoxetine in Overdose," *American Journal of Psychiatry* 147(August 1990): 1089.

Munoz, Ricardo, et al. "On the AHCPR Depression in Primary Care Guidelines," *American Psychologist* 49(1)(January 1994): 42–61.

Nakra, B. R., P. Szwabo, et al. "Mania Induced by Fluoxetine," Letter, *American Journal of Psychiatry* 146(11)(November 1989): 1515–16.

Narurkar, Vic. "Desipramine-Induced Blue-Gray Photosensitive Pigmentation," *JAMA* 270(July 7, 1993):28.

Nemeroff, Charles B., K. Ranga, et al. "Adrenal Gland Enlargement in Major Depression: A Computed Tomographic Study," *Archives of General Psychiatry* 49(May 1992): 384–87.

Ni, Y.G., and R. Miledi, "Blockage of 5HT2C serotonin receptors by fluoxetine (Prozac)," *Proceeds of the National Academy of Science USA* 94(March 4, 1997): 2036–40

Nolen-Hoeksema, Susan. *Sex Differences in Depression,* Stanford, CA: Stanford University Press, 1990.

Nulman, Irena, et al, "Neurodevelopment of children exposed in utero to antidepressant drugs," *New England Journal of Medicine* 336(1997): 258–62.

Nussar, Daniel. *Modell's Drugs in Current Use and New Drugs,* New York: Springer Publishing, 1993.

Ornstein, Robert, and C. Swencionis. *The Healing Brain: A Scientific Reader,* New York: Guilford Press, 1990.

Papolos, Demitri, and Janice Papolos. *Overcoming Depression,* New York: Harper Press, 1992.

Papp, L., and J. Gorman. "Suicidal Preoccupation During Fluoxetine Treatment," Letter, *American Journal of Psychiatry* 147(10)(October 1990): 1380–1.

Pappas, Nancy. "Skinny Pills," *Woman's Day* June 20, 1989, 37.

Paradis, Cynthia. "Nortriptyline and Weight Change in Depressed Patients Over 60," *JAMA* 269(January 6, 1993): 99.

Pastuszak, Anne, et al. "Pregnancy Outcome Following First-Trimester Exposure to Fluoxetine (Prozac)" *JAMA* 269(May 5, 1993): 2246–8.

Pharmaceutical Research and Manufacturers of America. "In Development: New Medicines for Mental Illness," *New Medicines in Development Series,* Washington, D.C.: May 1994.

1994 Physician's Desk Reference, Montvale, NJ: Medical Economics Data Production Co., 1994.

Piredda, S. G., and S. L. Rubinstein. "Hypomania Induced by Fluoxetine," *Biological Psychiatry* 32(1)(July 1, 1992): 107.

Pollack, M. H., and J. F. Rosenbaum. "Fluoxetine Treatment of Cocaine Abuse in Heroin Addicts," *Journal of Clinical Psychiatry* 52(1)(January 1991): 31–33.

Pigott, T. A., et al. "Controlled Comparisons of Clomipramine and Fluoxetine in the Treatment of Obsessive-Compulsive Disorder: Behavioral and Biological Results," *Archives of General Psychiatry* 48(9)(September 1991): 857–9.

Post, Robert M., and James C. Ballenger, eds. *Neurobiology of Mood Disorders,* Baltimore: Williams & Wilkins, 1984.

————, "Sensitization and Kindling Perspectives for the Course of Affective Illness: Toward a New Treatment with the Anticonvulsant Carbamazepine," *Pharmacopsychiatry* 23(1990): 3–17.

————, Gabriele S. Leverich, et al. "Carbamazepine Prophylaxis in Refractory Affective Disorders: A Focus on Long-term Follow-up," *Journal of Clinical Psychopharmacology* 10(1990): 318–27.

Potter, William. "The Pharmacologic Treatment of Depression," *The New England Journal of Medicine* 325(August 29, 1991): 633–42.

Preskorn, S. H, and M. Burke. "Somatic Therapy for Major Depressive Disorder: Selection of an Antidepressant," *Journal of Clinical Psychiatry* 53(9)(supp)(1992): 5–18.

————, J. H. Beber, et al. "Serious Adverse Effects of Combining Fluoxetine and Tricyclic Antidepressants," Letter, *American Journal of Psychiatry* 147(4)(April 1990): 532.

Prien, Robert F., and Alan J. Gelenberg. "Alternatives to Lithium for Preventive Treatment of Bipolar Disorder," *American Journal of Psychiatry* 146(1990): 840–8.

Prien, R. F. and D. J. Kupfer. "Continuation of Drug Therapy for Major Depressive Episodes: How Long Should It be Maintained?" *American Journal of Psychiatry* 143(1986): 18–23.

Quitkin, F. M., et al. "Phenelzine and Imipramine in Mood Reactive Depressives, Further Delineation of the Syndrome of Atypical Depression," *Archives of General Psychiatry* 46(9)(1989): 787–93.

Rakel, Robert, ed. *Conn's Current Therapy,* Philadelphia: W. B. Saunders, 1993.

Ramirez, L. C., J. Rosenstock, et al. "Effective Treatment of Bulimia with Fluoxetine, a Serotonin Uptake Inhibitor in a Patient with Type 1 Diabetes Mellitus," *The American Journal of Medicine* 88(May 1990): 540–1.

Reaves, John, and James B. Austin. *How to Find Help for a Troubled Kid: A Parent's Guide to Programs and Services for Adolescents*, New York: Henry Holt, 1990.

Reinherz, Helen Z., Geraldine Steward-Berghauer, et al. "The Relationship of Early Risk and Current Mediators to Depressive Symptomatology in Adolescence," *Journal of American Academy of Child and Adolescent Psychiatry* 28(1989): 942.

Reynolds, C.F. "Treatment of Depression in Special Populations," *Journal of Clinical Psychiatry* 53(9)(1992): 45–53.

Rinzler, Carol Ann. *Are You at Risk?* New York: Facts on File, 1991.

Robins, Lee N. and Darrel A. Regier, eds. *Psychiatric Disorders in America: The Epidemiologic Catchment Area Study*, New York: The Free Press, 1991.

Rosenfeld, Isadore. *The Best Treatment*, New York: Simon & Schuster, 1991.

Rosenthal, Norman E. *Seasons of the Mind*, New York: Bantam Books, 1990.

Rush, A.J. "Problems Associated with Diagnosis of Depression," *Journal of Clinical Psychiatry* 51(6)(1990): 15–22.

Sacra, Cheryl. "The New Cure-alls: Mood Lifters May Offer Handfuls of Hope for More Than Just Depression," *Health*, September 1990, 36–8.

Saline, Carol. "Don't Blame Prozac," *Philadelphia Magazine,* August 1991, 49–53.

Salzman, Carl. "The Current Status of Fluoxetine," *Neuropsychopharmacology* 7(4)(1992): 245–7.

Schad-Somers, Susanne P. *On Mood Swings: The Psychobiology of Elation and Depression,* New York: Plenum Press, 1990.

Schatzberg, A. F. "Dosing Strategies for Antidepressant Agents," *Journal of Clinical Psychiatry* 52(5)(supp)(1991): 14–20.

Schatzberg, A. F., and J. O. Cole. *Manual of Clinical Psychopharmacology* (2nd ed.), Washington, D.C.: American Psychiatric Press, 1991.

Schneier, F.R., et al. "Fluoxetine in Panic Disorders," *Journal of Clinical Psychopharmacology* 10(2)(1990): 119–21.

Schraml, F., G. Benedetti, et al. "Fluoxetine and Nortriptyline Combination Therapy," *American Journal of Psychiatry* 146(12)(December 1989): 1636–7.

Schuchman, Miriam, and Michael Wilkes. "Dramatic Progress Against Depression," *The New York Times Magazine,* October 7, 1990, S12.

Schulkin, Jay. "Melancholic Depression and the Hormones of Adversity: A Role for the Amygdala," *Current Directions in Psychological Science* 3(2)(April 1994): 41–4.

Schumer, Fran. "Bye-Bye, Blues: A New Wonder Drug for Depression," *New York,* December 18, 1989, 48–53.

Schwartz, John. "The Drug Did It: A Tough Sell in Court," *Newsweek,* April 1, 1991, 66.

"Scientology: The Cult of Greed," *Time,* May 6, 1991, 32–39.

Seligman, Martin. *Learned Optimism*, New York: Alfred Knopf, 1991.

Shapiro, Patricia Gottleib. *A Parents' Guide to Childhood and Adolescent Depression*, New York: Dell Publishing, 1994.

Simpson, S.G., and J. R. DePaulo. "Fluoxetine Treatment of Bipolar II Depression," *Journal of Clinical Psychopharmacology* 11(1)(1991): 52–54.

Simpson, G., and Kerrin White. "Monoamine Oxidase Inhibitors: Their Use in Clinical Practice," *Hospital and Community Psychiatry* 33(8)(August 1982): 615–6.

Skelly, Flora Johnson. "The Hype about Prozac: Here's How to Answer Your Patients' Questions and Improve Your Treatment of Chronic Depression," *American Medical News* 36(December 6, 1993): 13–15.

Slap, Gail, Dolores F. Vorters, et al. "Risk Factors for Attempted Suicide During Adolescence," *Pediatrics* 84(5)(November 1989): 769.

Sleek, Scott. "Could Prozac Replace Demand for Therapy?" *APA Monitor*, April 1994, 28.

Snyder, Solomon. *The New Biology of Mood*, New York: Pfizer, 1988.

Sobin, P., L. Schneider, and H. McDermott. "Fluoxetine in the Treatment of Agitated Dementia," Letter, *American Journal of Psychiatry* 146(12)(December 1989): 1636.

Stanford, S.C., "Prozac: panacea or puzzle?" *Trends in Pharmacological Science* 17(April 1996): 150–4.

Stark, R., and C. D. Hardison. "A Review of Multicenter Controlled Studies of Fluoxetine Versus Imipramine and Placebo in Outpatients with Major Depressive Disorder," *Journal of Clinical Psychiatry* 46(3)(1985): 53–58.

Stark, P., et al. "The Pharmacologic Profile of Fluoxetine," *Journal of Clinical Psychiatry* 46(1985): 7–13.

Stein, Dan J., et al. "Serotonergic Medications for Sexual Obsessions, Sexual Addictions and Paraphilias," *Journal of Clinical Psychiatry* 53(1992): 267–71.

Sternbach, H. "The Serotonin Syndrome," *American Journal of Psychiatry* 148(1991): 705–13.

Stinson, Stephen. "Psychoactive Drugs," *Chemical & Engineering News* 68 (October 15, 1990): 33–50.

Stokes, P. "The Changing Horizon in the Treatment of Depression: Scientific/Clinical Publication Overview," *Journal of Clinical Psychiatry* 52(5)(1991): 35–43.

Stone, Elizabeth. "Low Anxiety," *Mademoiselle* 99(January 1993): 46–7.

Styron, William. *Darkness Visible: A Memoir of Madness,* New York: Random House, 1990.

"Tailoring Treatment for Depression's Many Forms," *U.S. News & World Report,* March 5, 1990, 54–5.

Teicher, Martin, et al. "Emergence of Intense Suicidal Preoccupation During Fluoxetine Treatment," *American Journal of Psychiatry* 147(February 1990): 207–10.

Thayer, Robert. *The Biopsychology of Mood and Arousal,* New York: Oxford University Press, 1989.

Thomas, Patricia. "Sad Attack," *Harvard Health Letter,* October 1991, 1–4.

Thornton, Jim. "Pharm Aid: Ten New Medicines You Should Know About," *Men's Health*, October 1990, 73–77.

Toufexis, Anastasia. "Warnings About a Miracle Drug: Reports of Suicide Attempts in Prozac Users Raise Doubts About the Popular Antidepressant," *Time*, July 30, 1990, 54.

————. "The Personality Pill," *Time*, October 11, 1993, 61–2.

"Uplifting Pill," *Discover*, June 1991, 14–5.

U.S. Department of Health and Human Services. *Special Report on Depression Research*, Rockville, MD: 1983.

Venkataraman, S., et al. "Mania Associated with Fluoxetine Treatment in Adolescents," *Journal of the American Academy of Child and Adolescent Psychiatry* 31(2)(1992): 276–281.

Wartik, Nancy. "Depression: An Array of New Treatments Combats the Common Cold of Mental Illness," and "Manic-Depression: Not for Artists Only," *American Health*, December 1993, 39–42.

Wehr, T. A., and F. K. Goodwin. "Can Antidepressants Cause Mania and Worsen the Course of Affective Illness?" *American Journal of Psychiatry* 144(11)(1987): 1403–11.

Weintraub, Pamela. "Warning: Side Effects," *American Health*, April 1992, 36–7.

Wells, K. B., et al. "The Functioning and Well-Being of Depressed Patients: Results from the Medical Outcomes Study," *JAMA* 262(1989): 914–19.

Willensky, Diana. "Once in a Blue Mood," *American Health*, April 1991, 12.

Winokur, George. *Depression: The Facts.* New York: Oxford University Press, 1981.

————, et al, "Familial alcoholism in manic-depressive (bipolar) disease," *American Journal of Medical Genetics* 67(April 9, 1996): 197–201.

————, et al. "Further Distinctions Between Manic-Depressive Illness (Bipolar Disorder) and Primary Depressive Disorder (Unipolar Depression)," *American Journal of Psychiatry* 150(8)(August 1993): 1176–81.

Wirshing, W. C., T. Van Putten, et al. "Fluoxetine, Akathisia and Suicidality: Is There a Causal Connection?" Letter, *Archives of General Psychiatry* 49(1992): 580–1.

Wise, M. G., and S. E. Taylor. "Anxiety and Mood Disorders in Medically Ill Patients," *Journal of Clinical Psychiatry* 51(1)(1990): 27–32.

"Worried About Prozac," *Consumer Reports* 58(October 1993): 636.

Zajecka, John, et al. "The Role of Serotonin in Sexual Dysfunction: Fluoxetine-Associated Orgasm Dysfunction," *Journal of Clinical Psychiatry* 52(2)(February 1991): 66–8.

APPENDIX A

ORGANIZATIONS

Agency for Health Care Policy and Research
Executive Office Center
2101 East Jefferson St., Suite 501
Rockville, MD 20852
(800) 255-1708
(Provides general information on depression)

American Academy of Child and Adolescent Psychiatry
3615 Wisconsin Ave. NW
Washington, DC 20016
(Publishes free written material including "Facts for Families": 45 fact sheets covering issues of normal childhood and disorders)

Anxiety Disorders Association of America
PO Box 42514
Washington, DC 20015
(301) 231-5484

D/ART Program
(Depression/Awareness, Recognition, and Treatment)
National Institute of Mental Health
Rm 10-85
5600 Fishers Lane
Rockville, MD 20857
(800) 421-4211
(Provides free brochures about depression)

Depressed Anonymous
PO Box 17471
Louisville, KY 40217
Email: depanon@aol.com
(12-step program with newsletter, phone support, information and referrals, pen pals, workshops, conferences, and seminars. Information pack $5; D.A. manual $12.)

Depression and Related Affective Disorders Association
Meyer 3-181
600 N. Wolfe St.
Baltimore, MD 21287
(410) 955-4647
(410) 614-3241 (FAX)
(Provides education and information and supporting research, with newsletter, literature, phone support. Offers Young People's Outreach Project and Depression in the Workplace Project.)

Depression After Delivery
        PO Box 1282
        Morrisville, PA 19067
        (215) 295-3994
        (800) 944-4773 (to leave name and address for
        information to be sent)
        (Provides support and information for women who
        have postpartum depression, with telephone support
        in most states, newsletter [$30/year], group
        development guidelines, pen pals, and conferences.)

Emotions Anonymous
        PO Box 4245
        St. Paul, MN 55104
        (612) 647-9712
        (Telephone referrals to local chapters; publications
        available)

Federation of Families for Children's Mental Health
        (703) 684-7710
        (Parent-run volunteer group makes referrals to
        professionals and other parents throughout
        America)

GROW, Inc.
        2403 W. Springfield Ave.
        Box 3667
        Champaign, IL 61826
        (217) 352-6989
        FAX: (217) 352-8530
        (International 12-step mutual help program to
        provide know-how for avoiding and recovering

from a breakdown. Leadership training and
consultation to develop new groups; 143 groups in
IL, NJ, DE, RI and Australia, New Zealand, and
Ireland.)

National Alliance for the Mentally Ill
    2101 Wilson Blvd., Suite 302
    Arlington, VA 22201
    (703) 524-7600
    (800) 950-NAMI
    (703) 524-9094 (FAX)
    (Provides support groups for the families of the
    mentally ill; call the 800-number for location of a
    local group in your area)

National Committee on Youth Suicide Prevention
    67 Irving Place South
    New York, NY 10003
    (212) 532-2400

National Depressive and Manic-Depressive Association
    730 North Franklin St., Suite 501
    Chicago, IL 60610
    (312) 642-0049
    (800) 826-3632
    (312) 642-7243 (FAX)
    Online: http://www.ndmda.org
    (Offers information on depression and manic-
    depression, one-on-one support, referrals by
    phone; publications and audiotapes and videotapes.
    To locate a depressed-patient support group, call
    800-number between 8:30 A.M. and 5 P.M. CST)

National Foundation for Depressive Illness
    Suite 1528
    2 Penn Plaza
    PO Box 2257
    New York, NY 10116
    (212) 268-4260
    Hotline: (800) 239-1263 or (800) 248-4344
    (Recorded information about the symptoms and
    treatment of depression, how to obtain an infor-
    mation packet with a list of doctors who specialize
    in treating depression, and support groups in your
    area)

National Institute of Mental Health
    Public Inquiries Section
    Room 15 C-05
    5600 Fishers Lane
    Rockville, MD 20857
    (301) 443-4513
    U.S. Public Health Service
    PO Box 8547, Silver Spring, MD 20907
    (For a free copy of *Depression Is a Treatable Illness*,
    send a postcard asking for the "Depression Guide"
    to the above address)

National Mental Health Association
    1021 Prince St. or 1020 Prince St.
    Alexandria, VA 22314
    (800) 969-6642
    (Helpful publications on depression, list of local
    chapters for referral to support groups, home-based
    services, and professionals in your area)

National Organization for Seasonal Affective Disorder
(NOSAD)
> PO Box 40190
> Washington, DC 20016
> (Newsletter, support groups, information about SAD)

Obsessive-Compulsive Foundation, Inc.
> PO Box 70
> Milford, CT 06460
> (203) 878-5669 (day)
> (203) 874-3843 (recorded message)
> (203) 874-2826 (FAX)
> Online: http: //pages.prodigy.com/alwillen/ocf.html

Postpartum Support International
> 927 N. Kellog Ave.
> Santa Barbara, CA 93111
> (805) 967-7636 (daytime PST)
> (Provides education, advocacy, annual conference,
> encourages formation of support groups, phone
> support, referrals, literature, and newsletter).

Recovery, Inc.
802 N. Dearborn St.
Chicago, IL   60610
> (312) 337-5661
> (312) 337-5756 (FAX)
> Online: http://www.recovery-inc.com

(A community mental health organization that
offers a self-help method of will training with a
method of techniques for controlling behavior and
changing attitudes toward nervous symptoms,
anxiety depression, anger, and fear. Publishes
"Recovery Reporter" for members; provides
information on starting groups and leadership
training).

Research and Training Center on Family Support and
Children's Mental Health
    Regional Research Institute
    Portland State University
    PO Box 751
    Portland, OR 97207
    (800) 628-1696
    (Maintains computerized data base covering profes-
    sionals, organizations, and parent groups all over the
    United States; distributes literature on depression
    and other issues related to children's mental health)

Seasonal Studies
National Institute of Mental Health
    Building 10/4S-239
    9000 Rockville Pike
    Bethesda, MD 20892
    (Provides information on seasonal affective depres-
    sion and light therapy)

Society for Light Treatment and Biological Rhythms
PO Box 478
Wilsonville, OR 97070
(503) 694-2404
(Provides further information on seasonal affective
depression and light therapy)

Sun Net
PO Box 10606
Rockville, MD 20850
(Provides information on seasonal affective depres-
sion and light therapy)

How to Find Names of Local Mental-Health Professionals

Psychiatrists

American Academy of Child and Adolescent Psychiatry
3615 Wisconsin Ave. NW
Washington, DC 20016
(References to child and adolescent psychiatrists in local areas)

American Psychiatric Association
Division of Public Affairs
1400 K St. NW
Washington, DC 20005
(202) 682-6220
(Provides telephone numbers of district branches, which will refer to psychiatrist specialists in your area)

Psychologists

American Psychological Association
750 First Ave. NE
Washington, DC 20002-2424
(202) 336-5700
(Provides phone number of your state organization, which will make referrals to psychologists in your area)

APPENDIX C.

TWELVE-STEP PROGRAMS

All sorts of substances may be abused by depressed people trying to numb specific symptoms. Unfortunately, drugs and alcohol generally only worsen depression. Following is a list of self-help programs based on the well-known "12-step" method popularized by Alcoholics Anonymous.

Alcoholics Anonymous
    475 Riverside Drive
    PO Box 459
    Grand Central Station
    New York, NY 10163
    (212) 870-3400

Al-Anon Family Groups Headquarters, Inc.
    PO Box 862
    Midtown Station
    New York, NY 10018
    (800) 356-9996

A.R.T.S. Anonymous (Artists Recovering Through the Twelve Steps)
    PO Box 175
    Ansonia Station
    New York, NY 10023
    (212) 873-7075

Cocaine Anonymous
    3740 Overland Ave., Suite H
    Los Angeles, CA 90034
    (310) 559-5833

CoDependents Anonymous
    PO Box 33577
    Phoenix, AZ 85067
    (602) 277-7991 (in New York: 212-691-5199)

Emotions Anonymous
    PO Box 4245
    St. Paul, MN 55204
    (612) 647-9712

Gamblers Anonymous
    PO Box 17173
    Los Angeles, CA 90017

Narcotics Anonymous
    16155 Wyandotte St.
    PO Box 9999
    Van Nuys, CA 91409
    (818) 780-3951

Nicotine Anonymous
    PO Box 591777
    San Francisco, CA 94159
    (415) 750-0328

Overeaters Anonymous
    383 Van Ness Ave., Suite 1601
    Torrance, CA 90501

Sex Addicts Anonymous
    PO Box 70949
    Houston, TX 77270
    (713) 869-4902

Workaholics Anonymous
    PO Box 66150
    Los Angeles, CA 90066
    (310) 859-5804

APPENDIX D.

DEPRESSION LINKS ON THE WORLD WIDE WEB

Antidepressants

Antidepressant information
A site that gives detailed information on any drug name, together with its chemical formula and other technical information about dosage, side effects, and precautions. Search by brand name, manufacturer, or generic name.
http://www.druginfonet.com/index.html

Internet mental health: drugs
A relatively technical path that explains antidepressants, including the symptoms it is used to treat, how the drug works, when it shouldn't be used, warnings and guidelines for pregnancy, geriatrics, and drug interactions. The site also includes symptoms of overdose, dosage instructions, and the exact contents of the pill or liquid.
http://www.mentalhealth.com/p30.html

Medication listing and drug references
If you know the name of your medication (brand name or generic) you can find out all about it here. If more than one link is listed for a particular drug, then multiple drug references are found.
http://www.cmhc.com/guide/pro22.html

Rx list
Yet another source for drug information. Type in the name of any drug (brand or generic) and you'll receive a list of symptoms its designed to treat, side effects, adverse reactions and other information on related drugs.
http://www.rxlist.com

Prozac (fluoxetine)
Advice about precautions and side effects together with basic information about the drug.
http://www.mentalhealth.com/drug/p30-05.html

Prozac
Another relatively technical site that offers an extensive overview of the drug with hyperlinks to topics including "other antidepressants" and "usage in the elderly." Tables explain adverse effects in those with depression, bulimia, and obsessive-compulsive disorder.
http://www.fairlite.com/ocd/medications/prozac. html

Prozac threads
Dozens of threads from sci.med.pharmacy presented here.
http://pharminfo.com/drugdb/proz_arc.html

Bipolar Disorder (Manic Depression)

Bipolar disorder
Diagnostic criteria, treatments, suicide, news articles, list of books and movies, tips for tracing bipolar illness in your family.
http://www.frii.com/~parrot/bip.html

Bipolar disorder and alcoholism
A personal site dealing with bipolar disorder and alcoholism, with links to various alcohol abuse and bipolar resources.
http://www.sstar.com/jsharai/index.html

Bipolar disorder NIMH Gopher
gopher://zippy.nimh.nih.gov:70/00/documents/niimh/depression/bipolar

Bipolar disorder and significant others
Bipolar Significant Others is a private maiing list for those who are involved with someone suffering from bipolar affective disorder; the site contains advice from bipolar individuals and some basic information on the disorder.
http://graves.ipl.co.uk/~wiz/bp.html

Creativity and bipolar disorder
Articles and interviews about creativity and bipolar disorder.
http://www.i1.net/~juli/bipolar.html

Moodswing.org
The new home of the Bipolar Diorder FAQ, with a database of support groups, clinics, physicians, and psychologists who deal with manic depression. A bipolar disorder message board and regularly scheduled chat session are available, together with an online catalog of some of themost recommended books dealing with bipolar disorder.
http://www.moodswing.org/

The uni-bipolar disorders page (Duke University)
Contains the alt.support.depression FAQ and related
resources (including mailing lists, newsgroups, and web-
sites dedicated to mental health).
http://www.duke.edu/~ntd/depression.html

Depression—Children/Adolescents

Depression in children
Information to help educate parents and families about
psychiatric disorders affecting children and adolescents.
**http://www.psych.med.umich.edu/web/aacap/facts
Fam/depressd.html**

Manic depression in teens
Information to help educate parents and families about
teens and bipolar disorder.
**http://www.psych.med.umich.edu/web/aacp/facts
Fam/bipolar.html**

Teenage depression
Frequently asked questions about the rise of depression
during teenage years, with information to help detect suicide risk.
http://www.mentalhealth.com/mag1/p51-dp01.html

Depression—General

Depression
A discussion of the stages of depression from the onset to
the next level and beyond, with a list of warning behaviors

to help identify the problem, and suggestions for how to help a depressed friend.
gopher://gopher.uiuc.edu/00/UI/CSF/Coun/SHB /depress

Depression and mental health
An index of links with one-word descriptions that includes information such as symptoms of depression and questions and answers about depression.
http://drycas.club.cc.cmu.edu/~maire/depress.html

Depression Central
A page of links to depression, mood, and related disorders resources online maintained by a long-standing Internet psychiatrist Ivan Goldberg. You'll find lots of research and professional articles usually not included elsewhere.
http://www.psycom.net/depression.central.html

Depression FAQ
From the alt.support.depression newsgroup, this includes some information that has been added for non-U.S. readers; the entire FAQ can be downloaded.
http://avocado.pc.helsinki.fi/~janne/asdfaq/index. html

Depression home page
Resources divided into the areas of education, commercial, and miscellaneous.
http://www.isca.uiowa.edu/users/david- caropreso/depression.html

Depression Primer (Duke University)
A depression FAQ with general information (symptoms, causes, treatments, and so on). All files must be downloaded to be read.
http://www.duke.edu/%7Entd/DEPR/contents.html

Helpful facts about depression (NIMH gopher)
gopher://zippy.nimh.nih.gov/00/documents/nimh/depression/DepFact

Mood disorders
Information on a wide variety of problems from depression to seasonal affective disorder, with access to the depression FAQ (including information on causes, treatment, and medication with a depression primer outlining basic definitions and concepts). Other materials include articles on Prozac and other specific drugs.
http://www.avocado.pc.helsinki.fi/~janne/mood/mood.html

National Institutes of Mental Health Informational Brochures
Online access to brochures on bipolar disorder, facts about depressive illnesses, geriatric depression, suicide fact sheet, general information about depression, and suicide journal references.
http://www.nimh.nih.gov/publicat/bipolar.html

National Library of Medicine (gopher)
Information on depression and consumer information and how to screen for depression.

gopher://gopher.nim.nih.gov:70/11/hstat/ahcpr/de
press/TEMPgrp3

Online psychology
American Online's live Tuesday chat with Counselor
Kelly, who holds a master's degree in psychology from St.
Mary's.
American Online keyword "psych–Depression"
Understanding depression

*Overcoming depression and preventing suicide (State
University of New York/Buffalo)*
General information about depression including symptoms; this site includes the alt.support.depression FAQ.
**http://wings.buffalo.edu/student-
life/ccenter/Depression/**

Pendulum Resources
Comprehensive information source for bipolar disorder
and other mood disorders, including articles, online support groups, and so on.
http://www.pendulum.org/

Therapy FAQ
Everything you might wonder about starting psychotherapy from a client's perspective.
http://abulafia.st.hmc.edu/~mmiles/faq.html

Treatment of depression
Outline of general treatment guidelines which you may
want to understand for clinical depression and related

mood disorders, including psychotherapy, hospitalization, medications, ECT, and self-help.
http://www.cmhc.com/disorders/sx22t.html

Understanding depression
An overview of the causes and symptoms of depression, with guidelines to help you decide when and if you need to seek professional help.
http://www.odos.uiuc.edu/Counseling_Center/depress.html

Depression Resource Lists

Depression and mental health links
A small list of resources with one-line descriptions for each site.
http://drycas.club.cc.cmu.edu/%7Emaire/depress.html

Depression Home Page
Site listing an index to some of the more informative and useful web sites for depression broken up into four different depression categories (usergroups, education, commercial, and miscellaneous). Each offers a brief description about contents and usefulness.
http://www.geocities.com/Athens/Forum/9570/index.html

Depression Resource List
Depression resources online list with guide to available depression resources.
http://earth.execpc.com/~corbeau/

Internet Depression Resources Aquinas
A large listing of online depression resources as well as
links to personal stories of dealing with depression.
http://www.geocities.com/HotSprings/8376/

Mental health sources on the internet
Another list of resources, including the Beck Depression
Inventory and the best and worst things to say to someone who is depressed.
http://stripe.Colorado.EDU/~judy/depression/

Suicide resources on the Internet
Links to helpful mailing lists and common suicidal
resources online.
http://www.coil.com/~grohol/helpme.htm

Depression Screening Tests

Clinical depression screening test
This checklist can help determine if you or someone you
know is suffering from depression; results are given
online.
http://sandbox.xerox.com/pair/cw/testing.html

Online screening test (NYU psychiatry department)
Interactive quick screening test with online results
designed to give a preliminary idea about the presence of
mild to moderate depressive symptoms that indicate the
need for an evaluation by a mental health professional.
http://www.med.nyu.edu/Psych/screens/depres.html

Depression— Seasonal Affective Depression

SAD
This website presents the facts on Seasonal Affective
Depression from a clinic in Cambridge, England, together
with information on symptoms and treatments, a product
catalog, and research abstracts.
http://www.outsidein.co.uk/bodyclock/sadinfo.html

*Seasonal Affective Disorder (University of British
Columbia)*
Maintained by a branch of the university's psychiatry project, this site provides information on symptoms, treatments, and suggested readings for SAD.
http://www.psychiatry.ubc.ca/mood/md_sad.html

Self-Help Groups

Depressed Anonymous
The email contact for this international 12-step group
that aims to help depressed people.
depanon@aol.com

Depression Alliance
The largest charity in Britain run by and for sufferers of
depression and those who love them. This site offers text
of current leaflets, book lists, selections from the newsletter, and some relevant links.
http://www.gn.apc.org/da/

Depression and Related Affective Disorders Association
Web site for the DRADA at Johns Hopkins University
School of Medicine, with selected articles from DRDA's

quarterly, information on support services programs, recommended books and videos, and related resources on the Internet. DRADA works with the psychiatry department at Johns Hopkins to ensure its materials are medically accurate and up to date.
http://infonet.welch.jhu.edu/departments/dradadefault/

National Depressive and Manic-Depressive Association
The website for this national organization provides public education on the biochemical nature of depressive and bipolar illnesses. Several educational booklets are available at this site, including one for dealing with depressed loved ones. Special sections are devoted to suicide and to adolescents. National DMDA membership, program, and chapter information are included.
http://www.ndmda.org

National Foundation for Depressive Illness, Inc.
Provides public and professional information about affective disorders, treatment, and the need for more research.
http://www.depression.org/

Recovery, Inc.
Website for this international community mental health organization offers a self-help method of will training to help control depression.
http://www.recovery-inc.com

The Samaritans
A non-religious charity offering emotional support to the suicidal; the service is available via email from

Cheltenham, England, and can be reached from anywhere with Internet access. Trained volunteers read and reply to mail once a day, every day of the year.
http://www.samaritans.org.uk/

Suicide

Suicide: Read this first
Conversations and writings for suicidal persons, with a few simple prevention materials and links to other helpful sites.
http://www.geocities.com/RainForest/1801/suicide1.html

Suicide prevention
This website for the Suicide Awareness, Voices of Education (SAVE) organization offers detailed information about identifying, treating, and stablilizing depression to avoid suicide, common statistics, symptoms of depression, a book list, and more..
http://www.save.org

Suicide counseling via email
For anyone contemplating suicide, the Samaritans (a 40-year-old counseling group in the United Kingdom) provides service via email. Trained volunteers answer requests for information using the name "Jo." Those requesting information will receive the FAQ file containing directions about anonymously emailing the Samaritans.
Email: jo@samaritans.org

Suicide FAQ
This FAQ addresses common problems in caring for a depressed friend or family member.
http://www.lib.ox.ac.uk/internet/news/faq/archive/suicide.info.html

Suicide prevention brochure
An essay on prevention designed for the friend or loved one of a potential suicide victim, with suggestions for dealing with the situation.
gopher://gopher.uiuc.edu:70/00/UI/CSF/Coun/SHB/suiprev

Suicide prevention
A brochure that tries to help identify those at risk for suicide, listing danger signals (including words and actions to watch for), and facts and statistics that dispel some myths about suicide.
http://www.odos.uiuc.edu/Counseling_Center/suiprev.html

Newsgroups

alt.support.depression (depression and mood disorders)
alt.support.depression.manic (manic depression and
   bipolar disorders)
alt.support.depression.seasonal (seasonal affective
   disorder, or SAD)
sci.med.psychobiology (dialog and news in psychiatry and
   psychobiology)
sci.psychology.misc (general discussion of psychology)
sci.psychology.psychotherapy (practice of psychotherapy)

soc.support.depression.crisis (personal crisis situations)
soc.support.depression.family (coping with depressed
  people)
soc.support.depression.manic (bipolar (manic depression)
soc.support.depression.misc (depression and mood
  disorders)
soc.support.depression.seasonal (seasonal affective
  disorder, or SAD)
soc.support.depression.treatment (treatments of
  depression)

Mailing Lists

bipolar disorder (manic depression)
majordomo@ucar.edu

depression and bipolar disorder
walkers-request@world.std.com

depression, Christian-oriented
hub@xc.org

partners and family of depressed people
majordomo@truespectra.com

suicide support
suicide-support-request@research.canon.com.au

suicide survivors
suicide-survivors-request@research.canon.com.au

Index